Introductory Medicine for Engineers

Basic medical knowledge, procedures and culture

Introductory Medicine for Engineers

Basic medical knowledge, procedures and culture

Edited By
Yi Wang, PhD
Departments of Biomedical Engineering and Radiology
Cornell University, New York
USA

First printing, 2015

ISBN:151190481X

Library of Congress Cataloging-in-Publication applied for.

This book is dedicated to the clinicians at Weill Cornell Medical College who have volunteered their precious time in the past years to serve as mentors for the Clinical Summer Immersion for Biomedical Engineering PhD Students, particularly to William W. Frayer MD.

Any medical center can be overwhelming and stressful. It is typically crowded with sick patients and their concerned family and friends, busy physicians trying to cure patients, and nurses, technicians, receptionists and administrators supporting physicians to care for patients. It is fundamentally to provide clinical diagnosis and treatment, which require understanding of the complex human body in health and disease conditions. Modern medicine always involve complicated equipment to perform diagnostic tests and deliver therapies. The developments of these medical devices depend on engineers and their collaborations with physicians. However, engineering curriculum generally does not include medicine, leaving a critical gap between engineers and physicians that hinders the advancement of healthcare technology.

This concise book aims to fill this gap between engineers and physicians. It is designed to provide a quick introduction to medicine for engineering students want to learn about the basics of medicine and its practice, concepts, and customs. The materials of the book largely come from the Clinical Summer Immersion for Biomedical Engineering PhD Students, which has been running in the past decade at Weill Medical College of Cornell University. The focus of this concise book is on introduction, including general cultures and customs of a hospital, medical terminology, medical imaging as a major diagnostic tool, surgical devices, basic surgical treatment, process of medicine exemplified by the treatment of arthritis, basic pharmaceuticals.

We hope that this book will help engineers gain knowledge of a clinical medical setting and confidence to work in or interface with such a setting. We further hope that this book may help engineers to find that the field of healthcare technology innovation is intellectually stimulating and gratifying.

ACKNOWLEDGEMENTS

We are very grateful to Bill Frayer, who served many years prior to his recent retirement as a co-director of Cornell's Clinical Summer Immersion program and helped tremendously with hospital culture and customs and process of medicine. We are very thankful to Bill Olbricht, who served as the PI on Cornell's Med into Grad Initiative program funded by Howard Hughes Medical Institute, which helps funding the writing of this book.

We thank physicians who have served as clinician mentors in Cornell's Clinical Summer Immersion program: Bessey, Palmer "Joe"; Boockvar, John; Bostrom, Mathias ; Bykerk, Vivian; Bush Jr., Harry; Cesarman, Ethel; Cross, Michael; Cunningham, Matthew; Ebben, Matthew; Farmer, Brenna; Gauthier, Susan; Girardi, Leonard; Gobin, Pierre; Goodman, Susan; Grant, Robert; Greenfield, Jeff; Gupta, Ajay; Hartl, Roger; Healey, John; Kamel, Hooman; Kaplitt, Michael; Kapur, Sandip; Kennedy, John; Lane, Joseph M.; Lavi, Ehud; Lee, Sang; Leifer, Dana; McKinsey, Scarlett; Miller, Andy; Lockshin, Michael; Milsom, Jeffrey ; Nanus, David; Pannullo, Susan; Potter, Hollis; Prince, Martin; Rodeo, Scott; Rosenblatt, Mark; Salemi, Arash ; Schafer, Andrew; Scherr, Douglas; Schwartz, Ted; Shah, Manish ; Shin, Sandra; Shou, Jianj; Silver, Richard; Souweidane, Mark; Spector, Jason; Spigland, Nitsana; Stieg, Phil; Te, Alexis; Tsiouris, John; Vahdat, Linda; Weinsaft, Jonathan; Wong, Chui.

We thank Mark Williams for editing assistance.

CONTRIBUTORS

Andrea Gardner,
PhD candidate
Biomedical Engineering,
Cornell University, Ithaca, NY

Jason Guss,
PhD candidate
Biomedical Engineering,
Cornell University, Ithaca, NY

Ilhami Kovalikaya, MD,
Professor
Radiology,
Weill Cornell Medical College,
New York, NY

Zhe Liu,
PhD candidate
Biomedical Engineering,
Cornell University, Ithaca, NY
Department of Radiology,
Weill Cornell Medical College,
New York, NY

Andrew J. Luzzi
Department of Radiology,
Weill Cornell Medical College,
New York, NY

Frank A. Luzzi, MD,
Chief
Otolaryngology
Northwest Ear Nose Throat Specs,
Torrington, CT

Martin R. Prince, MD, PhD,
Professor
Radiology,
Weill Cornell Medical College,
Professor
Radiology,
Columbia University College of
Physicians and Surgeons,
New York, NY

Yi Wang, PhD,
Professor
Biomedical Engineering,
Cornell University, Ithaca, NY
Faculty Distinguished
Professorship in
Radiology
Weill Cornell Medical College,
New York, NY

TABLE OF CONTENTS

CHAPTER 1

WHAT'S THE USE FOR BIOMEDICAL ENGINEERS TO LEARN ABOUT CLINICAL PRACTICE?

Yi Wang, PhD

What use is it for biomedical engineers to learn about clinical practice? This may be the first and one of most important questions for an engineering student or a practicing engineer interested in this book. This question can be partially addressed by examining the very definition of biomedical engineering (BME). I will use my experience as an engineer working on medical imaging technology to demonstrate how important it is for biomedical engineers to have some knowledge about medicine and clinical practice.

1.1   BIOMEDICAL ENGINEERING (BME) AND MEDICINE

Clinicians, scientists, and engineers are all integral parts of the healthcare team and must work cooperatively in the long, challenging battle against disease. The challenges in translating basic research advances in life sciences from laboratory test tubes and mice to the clinical arena are formidable because test tubes and mice, though instrumental for scientific investigation, cannot fully replicate human disease. To address these challenges, the discipline of biomedical engineering (BME) has been formed to integrate engineering with life sciences and medicine. BME's objective is to develop medical technology and subsequently improve medical care.

Medical technology created to monitor, prevent, diagnose, control and cure a growing number of health conditions has greatly influenced medical practice and healthcare outcomes. Medical technology has become an integral and significant component of healthcare and has permeated into all major aspects of medical practice, including surgical procedures (angioplasty, joint replacements, organ transplants), diagnostic tests (laboratory tests, biopsies, imaging), drugs (biologic agents, pharmaceutics, vaccines), interventional devices (implantable defibrillators, stents, prosthetics) and support systems (electronic medical records and telemedicine). In fact, MRI (magnetic resonance imaging) and CT (computed tomography) scanning are regarded as the top medical innovations in recent times (Fuchs VR, Sox HC,

Physicians' Views Of The Relative Importance Of Thirty Medical Innovations, Health Affair, 20(5): 30-42, 2001).

In order for biomedical engineers to be effective in their endeavor of improving medical technology, they must not only understand basic biological and engineering sciences, but also comprehend the clinical requirements of both patients and clinicians and the impact BME has on healthcare and society. Clinical experiences reveal how diseases affect patients, how diseases are diagnosed and treated in medical practice, how medical technologies are invented, disseminated and utilized in healthcare facilities, and how medical technologies influence medical practice, the economy and society.

1.2   GAP BETWEEN INTENSE AND FOCUSED ENGINEERING STUDY AND BUSY CLINICAL PRACTICE

I did my PhD study on MRI. Though we did research on the MRI scanners in the hospital and our office was in the hospital, we never spent time in the reading room to see how radiologists made diagnoses from MRI images. We were too focused on learning the complex spin dynamics underlying MRI and too busy with coding and testing new pulse sequences. Few of the new pulse sequences that we were developing would show enough promise to warrant the evaluation of the sequences by radiologists in a clinical setting. Consequently, very few of the PhD students working on MRI actually worked closely with radiologists.

Like all clinicians, radiologists are very busy. I do recall peeking into a reading room. It was dimly lit so that radiologists could read the films displaced on the huge panel of light boxes (nowadays, the reading room is full of large monitors that display the digital images, but it is still dim.) Radiologists were busy flipping through panels of images and making dictations, and interrupting them in order to gain their attention was difficult and made me feel uncomfortable. Though we were testing pulse sequences on the same MRI scanners that were being used in clinical practice, we gained access to the scanners only after the clinical hours.

My four years of PhD thesis work on developing MRI to image coronary arteries went by very quickly. Coronary MRI continues to challenge researchers and is still in the investigational stage 20 years after I wrote my thesis. Despite having completed four years of study, I did not have the chance to work with clinicians in evaluating my pulse sequence for imaging coronary arteries and I did not learn much about the use of MRI in clinical practice.

1.3 CLINICAL PRACTICE IS A FERTILE GROUND FOR IDEAS OF TECHNICAL INNOVATIONS

Following the completion of my PhD in early 1994, I continued to work on the development of coronary MRI in my postdoctoral training. Imaging the moving coronary arteries was a challenge that opened opportunities for many technical innovations. I took these opportunities, came up with many technical improvements, and generated many papers. However, my efforts could not make coronary MRI sufficiently robust for clinical practice. I was not sure what to do next in my research, which was quite disturbing for a postdoc looking for a job. To determine if I should stay in MRI, I needed to know something about the MRI market. I needed to know how MRI was used in clinical practice.

Fortunately, my postdoc advisor, Dr. Richard Ehman, is a great clinician, in addition to being a first rate physicist. Because of Dr. Ehman, I was able to spend some time in the radiology reading room. I was amazed by the many diseases, images, and the empirical or semi-empirical connections between them. While I admired radiologists' good memory, I realized that for a technique to be used in clinical practice, it has to be highly reproducible. A good idea that leads to a cute paper is not enough; a great idea is one that works in practice.

My brief exposure to the radiology reading room led me to reassess my own research work. Coronary MRI was a prime area for technical innovation, but what could bridge the gap between its research development and its incorporation in the clinic? Seeing this gap was both refreshing and frightening. The refreshing aspect would later define one R01 (a major type of NIH grants) project on coronary MRI when I became an independent investigator. The frightening aspect would prompt me to diversify applications of techniques developed by my research, such as imaging arteries other than coronary arteries, which would later define another R01 project. I would like to relate specific stories on how I developed time-resolved imaging and bolus chase techniques for contrast enhanced magnetic resonance angiography (CEMRA). CEMRA is a major method to image blood vessels in MRI without x-ray radiation. However, CEMRA faced two major problems in clinical problems: 1) clinicians had to guess the time of contrast arriving at a targeted body part to start imaging, but varieties in diseases make timing-guess difficult and CEMRA quality suffers with mistiming; 2) different body parts had to be imaged by repositioning the patients and repeating contrast injection.

The story of time-resolved imaging for CEMRA. The tail end of the second year of my postdoctoral training was soon upon me, and I began to actively explore my job options. During my visits to reading rooms, I was very fortunate to meet with Dr. John Huston, a great neuroradiologist who was interested in MRI research. Dr. Huston performs neuro interventional procedures, such as placing stents to open carotid arteries, in addition to reading MRIs. Dr. Huston allowed me to observe his next interventional case. Though the sight of blood at the femoral artery puncture made me light-headed, I was fascinated by the use of imaging in guiding therapy, in addition to imaging based diagnosis. It was also amazing to see the speed of x-ray imaging (relative to MRI) and to witness clinicians' skill in performing treatment under limited anatomical information in x-ray fluoroscopy. Blood vessels were imaged using x-ray digital subtraction angiography (DSA), which was invented by my PhD thesis advisor, Prof. Charles Mistretta. DSA is based on serial or time-resolved imaging of a body part to capture contrast bolus passing through the vasculature. The subtraction of contrast enhanced 2D images (thick slab or projection without resolution along depth) by a mask image acquired prior to contrast arrival generates an image of the vessels containing contrast agent. Right after my trip to the interventional radiology suite with Dr. Huston, I realized that the same thing could be done in CEMRA to address the mistiming problem. As I looked into x-ray angiography more, I also realized that the moving table used in x-ray fluoroscopy to do bolus chase angiography in the lower extremity could be borrowed for MRI, which is the idea of the multi-station-stepping-table as described below. Immediately, I started to develop a time-resolved imaging approach for CEMRA, as well as mask subtraction. Soon, we published a paper on magnetic resonance digital subtraction angiography (MRDSA). MRDSA ushered in the field of time-resolved CEMRA that remains to be active for both clinical practice and scientific research.

The story of the multi-station-stepping-table (MSST) platform in MRI and bolus chase CEMRA. Near the end of my postdoc, I felt that I could do a lot in improving MRI for clinical practice and I could realize this by developing my own MRI research program in an academic center. In 1997, I started my own research lab at Cornell University. I worked closely with interventional radiologists Drs. Neil Khilnani and David Trost to develop the MSST platform for MRI to address the problem that many fields-of-view are needed to image a long territory, such as in the lower extremity. This MSST solution was particularly useful for imaging arteries in the legs following a single contrast bolus. Soon we developed the bolus chase CEMRA using MSST to image peripheral arteries from feet to abdomen, in a manner similar to x-ray bolus chase angiography. This was a very fruitful pursuit, as we published many papers and received an R01 grant. We were awarded several patents but they were licensed very cheaply. Still, it was gratifying to see our work become commercial products (Siemens' total imaging matrix, TIM) and be used in routine clinical practice.

1.4   THE IMPACT OF A BIOMEDICAL ENGINEERING IDEA HAS TO BE ASSESSED IN CLINICAL PRACTICE

My career as a biomedical imaging engineer in an academic setting has benefited tremendously from collaborating with clinicians: I would learn about the unmet clinical needs and think about technical solutions to address these unmet needs; I would learn different ways to do things and incorporate them into what I was doing. This point has been illustrated in my stories as described above. I would like to exemplify another need for biomedical engineers to work with clinicians by evaluating and disseminating information about developed technology. Bringing new techniques to clinical practice may help improve patient care and is critical for generating a societal impact.

The issue of improving patient care with new technology is quite complex, involving many players besides engineers. Clinicians are needed to do clinical trials to demonstrate efficacy; business people are needed to invest into the product development and marketing; bureaucrats and lawyers are involved in FDA approval. Perhaps the most important initial step is obtaining preliminary clinical data to demonstrate the clinical utility of a new technology. When a new technique is developed specifically to address an unmet need in clinical practice, the clinical utility of the new technique is well defined, and clinicians are eager to perform evaluation to find out how much the new technique will improve their practice. Often we engineers may come up with ideas from insights in technologies, not from responding to unmet clinical needs. There are many cases where the clinical utilities are not clearly defined, and engineers have to actively seek out clinicians to identify any clinical use of their technologies.

To illustrate the necessity of engineers reaching out to clinicians to establish clinical utilities, I shall describe one example from my own experience.

Recently, my lab has been working on solving the inverse problem from magnetic field to tissue magnetic susceptibility. The magnetic field can be estimated from MRI data. Tissue magnetic susceptibility reflects molecular electron polarization, an important piece of molecular information of the tissue, in the magnetic field of MRI. This field-to-susceptibility inverse problem is a fundamental problem in physics that has not been solved. We feel fortunate to have found an important physics problem to work on and we are excited that this problem is solvable in the context of MRI. About 5 years ago (2010), we came up the Bayesian approach with a reasonable solution and published our technique as quantitative susceptibility mapping (QSM). How would QSM benefit patient care? We have been struggling with this question ever since. QSM may be used to improve hemorrhage diagnosis. QSM may be used to improve visualization of targets in deep brain stimulation. QSM may be used to study multiple sclerosis. QSM may be used to assess brain iron accumulation that is associated with neurodegeneration in ailments such as Parkinson's disease and Alzheimer's disease. We are actively working with neurologists and surgeons to identify the clinical efficacy of QSM.

1.5 THE PURPOSE OF THIS BOOK IS TO HELP BRIDGE THE GAP BETWEEN ENGINEERS AND CLINICIANS

Getting your feet into the door of a medical center and approaching busy clinicians can be difficult and intimidating, as I experienced initially. This problem is partly caused by the engineer's lack of knowledge about medical practice. Here we try to ease this problem for engineers by introducing the basic clinical procedures, vocabulary, and culture.

CHAPTER 2

CULTURES AND CUSTOMS IN THE HOSPITAL, IMMERSION EXPERIENCE OF A BME STUDENT

Andrea Gardner

Being immersed in a hospital setting for the first time can be an intimidating experience for anyone. Hospitals have rigid organizational structure and strict policies that are not always immediately apparent to an unexperienced bystander. Many biomedical engineers have never had any significant clinical experience and, though some may feel perfectly comfortable and confident with the idea of being immersed in a hospital setting, others may not. Collaboration between biomedical engineers and clinicians is critical to the advancement of medical technology. For this reason, the clinical exposure of engineers is of utmost importance. This chapter hopes to educate biomedical engineers about the cultures and customs of a hospital so that they may feel more comfortable in a clinical setting and so that collaboration between engineers and clinicians, and the idea generation which hopefully results, may be fostered.

2.1   MEDICAL HIERARCHIES

Upon entering a hospital, one of the most difficult aspects of medical practice to grasp is the medical hierarchy and determining who is in charge. Everyone is dressed in white coats or scrubs and they are all referred to as doctors. However, engrained in the medical education system is a hierarchy, in which doctors start as medical students and may work their way up the pyramid. The main roles seen in a teaching hospital in the US are depicted in Fig.2.1.

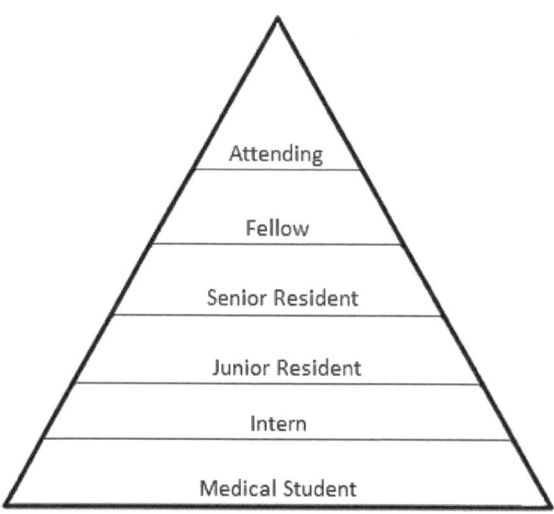

Fig.2.1. Hierarchy of staff in the medical profession.

- A medical student, or med student, is a person who is still enrolled in a graduate medical program and has not yet earned their MD.
- An intern is a graduate of medical school, but does not yet have a license to practice unsupervised clinical medicine. Often, an internship is part of a multi-year residency, in which residents in their first year are referred to as interns. Upon completion of the one-year internship or first year of residency, the doctor may practice as a general practitioner without supervision.
- A medical resident is someone who holds a medical degree and wishes to pursue training in a specialty field. Residencies can last 3 to 7 years depending on the specialty, for example, a residency in emergency medicine averages around 3 years, while a residency in urology averages around 5 years. Most hospitals require that the attending physician supervise all medical decisions made by residents.
- A junior resident is someone who is in the first half of his or her residency.
- A senior resident is someone who is in the second half of his or her residency. Senior residents are often given more responsibility and independence within the hospital than junior residents.
- A fellow is someone who has completed their residency program and obtained medical license and seeks training in a sub-specialty through a fellowship. Examples of what someone may pursue as a fellowship include: cardiology, endocrinology, immunology, neonatology, oncology, and more. Completion of a fellowship would allow that doctor to practice that sub-specialty without supervision.
- The attending physician must have completed a residency program and often has fellowship training as well. The attending physician is responsible for all aspects of patient care in his or her ward, often

through supervisory and teaching interactions with residents, interns, and medical students.

2.2   INTERACTING WITH DOCTORS

The hierarchy of graduate medical education is well established, and students of the medical education system are accustomed to respecting those further along, but how should engineers approach this unfamiliar educational pyramid?

First, one must never forget that doctors, just like patients, nurses, yourself, and everyone else in the world, are just people. And as with everyone in the world, people have different personality types, different experiences, and different perspectives that are constantly influencing actions and reactions to situations. Still, though, some general behavioral advice on how to act when working with doctors may be helpful.

Step 1: Introduction yourself:
"Hi, I'm Andrea, I'm a visiting biomedical engineering student from Cornell Ithaca."

When meeting someone with a hospital badge, first introduce yourself and explain your role, then allow them to introduce themselves. If it is not apparent by their badge or their introduction, you can ask what their role is. Every person in every role in the hospital, not just doctors, can help add perspective and understanding to your experience. Make sure to take complete advantage of the vast knowledge hiding in the minds of those around you.

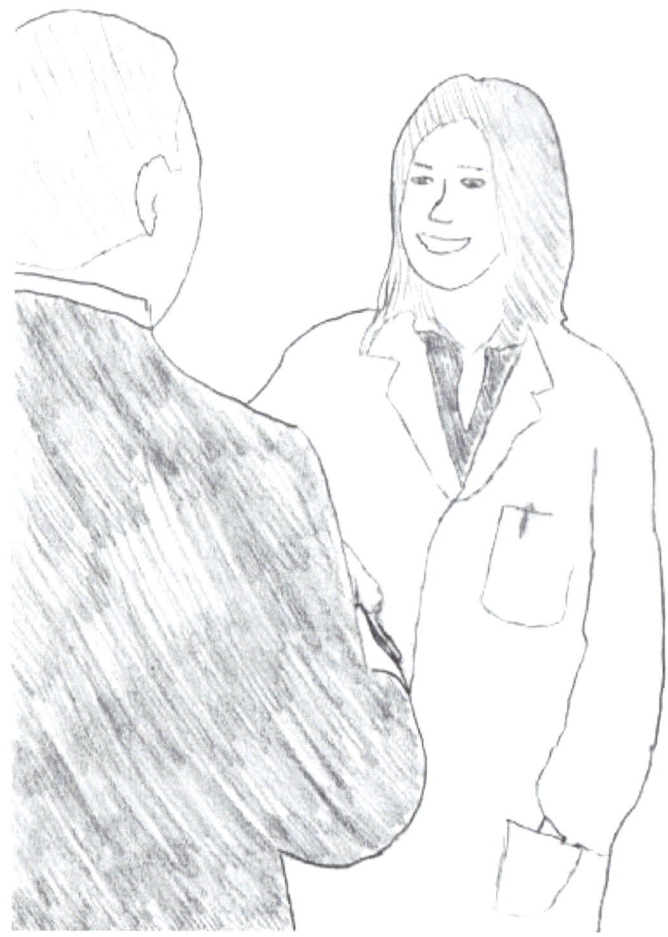

Fig.2.2. Say Hi!

Step 2: Give them a reason to interact with you

"As part of my graduate research, I design and build low-cost medical equipment, but I've never really seen medicine in action. I'd love to watch how you use tools to interact with patients to gain that perspective. Additionally, if you have any complaints about current tools or lack of tools, we might be able to work together to design something new."

Most doctors gladly disseminate their knowledge to others in their profession and many doctors strive to educate more than just their peers, but what can you do if you are placed with a doctor who does not see the use in sharing knowledge with you, the observer?

In this case, it is sometimes helpful to try to learn from the residents. Residents are known for being more open, but even residents can sometimes overlook the importance of you being in the room.

An engineer is at the hospital to observe and learn about the clinical practice of medicine and areas of potential improvement. This is made more difficult if the medical experts at the hospital are unwilling to share their knowledge. It can be helpful to mention that, as an engineer, you plan to strive to improve various aspects of health care through technological advancement and innovation. The intent of this is to establish your value as both an intelligent and competent professional and an individual whose goal is to improve something that could be important to the doctor.

If, despite your best efforts, you cannot find a physician, resident, or other healthcare professional to share their knowledge and experiences, make the best of your situation. Attempting to force others to want to interact with you will lead to a negative experience for both you and those with whom you are working. Instead, acknowledge the situation, attempt to absorb as much of the experience as you can, and in the future look for other healthcare workers who may be more willing to indulge your intellectual curiosities.

Step 3: Joining rounds and determining what makes a good question

Doctors perform rounds together to keep each other updated on each patient. Rounds can vary significantly from department to department. Often radiology rounds consist of a gathering of doctors around a table discussing each patient's symptoms while viewing that patient's x-ray, CT, or MRI at the front of the room. On the contrary, emergency department rounds happen during shift handoffs and the doctors physically meet with each patient as a group and try to formulate a plan. What both of these scenarios have in common is that during rounds, a single patient is focused upon and discussed amongst multiple doctors before moving onto the next patient. Medicine is often a top-down process, with the attending always supervising and directing patient care, but rounds give an opportunity for more democratic discussions to occur between doctors of all training levels.

Joining rounds can be intimidating (Fig.2.2). If you are not prepared, it can feel like you are being thrown case study after case study and barely given enough time to hunt for the recognizable Latin or Greek roots in the first symptom listed before the discussion of the next case begins.

Before going on rounds, doctors print out patient cheat sheets that show abbreviated notes of each patient's time in the hospital, which include the patient's primary condition, current medications, and intake date. You are allowed to request a copy of this information so long as you protect it in accordance with the federal Health Insurance Portability and Accountability Act of 1996 (HIPAA). Getting to rounds early will allow you to review the patient information and discover any questions that can be more easily answered ahead of time. For example, instead of getting lost in words during rounds, one of the residents or a discreet Internet search can quickly tell you that xerostomiath is simply dry mouth.

This applies outside of rounds as well, but especially during rounds: always carry a pocket sized notebook and a pen. Even if you prepare as much as possible, doctors may still be throwing around terminology and prescribing procedures and treatments of which you have never heard. Write it all down, as this will allow you to ask or look up questions later.

If the day is slow, the physicians may welcome questions from you during rounds. However, typically rounds are chaotic and it can be very hard to get a word in on the side. If you do find an opportunity to ask a question, you want to make sure it is a good one.

Only you can determine which question to ask in order to get the most out of your experience, but here are some aspects of consideration to help determine if a question is worth asking during rounds:

1) Can I look this up on the Internet later?
   If the answer is yes, it is probably not worth asking during hectic rounds.

2) Is it possible that asking this question in front of the patient could make the patient uncomfortable or distressed?
   If your answer is even maybe, you should save your question for later when you are not within hearing range of the patient.

3) Will knowing the answer to this right now change my experience?
   While I was rounding in the pediatric ICU, I kept hearing a word I did not know over and over again. I tried to write it down, but was not able to spell what I was hearing. Though I was embarrassed to ask because of how often they were using the word, asking what it meant for someone to be tachypneic and receiving an answer (tachypnea: rapid breathing) exponentially increased my understanding of each patients' condition from that point forward and allowed me to focus on the people in front of me rather than a word.

4) Could asking this question potentially shift the doctors' perspective in a way that would benefit the patient?

Just because you do not have years of medical training does not mean you should not listen to your intuition. Maybe you read a paper once about a rare disease that the patient in front of you seems to fit. When framing the question of whether or not the doctors have already looked into a certain disease or treatment, always make the humble assumption that they have already thought of it. Even if they have already thought of it, discussion on why they do not believe a patient has a particular disease may encourage follow-up testing or at least interesting discussion within the group.

2.3   INTERACTING WITH PATIENTS

Conversing with patients, obviously in a way that does not impede their care, can be enriching for both you and the patient. As most engineers have never been given the opportunity to converse with patients on a daily basis, here are some general guidelines on how to interact with those who are being treated in a hospital.

Step 1: Introduce Yourself
"Hi Mr. Johnson, my name is Andrea, I'm a biomedical engineering graduate student."

Be honest and open about your position as a graduate student observer. Sometimes they will even be curious and want to learn more about your program.

If the patient will be conscious for the procedure, you should get their permission for you to ask questions to the doctor performing the procedure as it is done. Questions, or even the answers to your questions, may make the patient feel anxious or uncomfortable. If the patient prefers that you not ask questions during the procedure, jot down your questions in a notebook and ask the attending physician or residents later.

Step 2: Get to Know the Patient and Connect with Them
"So, Mr. Johnson, tell me a little more about yourself, where are you from?"

Talking to patients can be difficult without knowing their background and what might trigger upset, so try to stick to neutral subjects. You can ask how they are doing, but because they are in a hospital their response may be negative. Not every patient will have friends and family waiting for them, so wait until they bring up people in their life before asking about family. A more neutral question you can start with is "Where are you from?" Everyone has a story to tell and if the patient is in the mood for talking, this is a good place to start. If the patient prefers not to talk, do not try to force it. Just let them know that you are around if they need anything.

Step 3: Do something about it!
"Hey Tom, Mr. Johnson is really uncomfortable, do you think you can help him shift when you get a chance? Thanks so much!"

In non-life threatening cases, you, as an observer, should be adhering to a hands-off policy. You can still help the patient, though, if he or she needs anything by signaling for the person who can help. For example, if the patient needs to shift in the bed or manipulate the IV, listen and then find a nurse to care for the patient.

Additionally, July and August can be an especially difficult time to be a patient. This is the time in which new residents and fellows show up and are learning the ropes from the senior physicians. A new resident may be performing the procedure and the attending may be yelling orders from across the room. I have seen a patient's heart rate increase by 30bpm, as she laid there with the junior resident yelling back to the attending while repositioning the chest tube over and over again. In times like these, go back to step 2. Talk to the patient and take their mind off of what is happening.

Step 4: Keep them Informed
"Good to see you again, Mr. Johnson, just wanted to let you know that your CT scan uploaded to the computers and we're just waiting for a read from the radiologist now. Hopefully we'll have some updates for you soon!"

If your patient or the patient's family is waiting on results, do your best to keep them informed! Again, you can remind them that you have little authority to take action as a student, but most of the time the patient and/or family will just be happy to hear that someone is thinking about them and that they are not getting lost in the medical ether. This step is especially important in busy areas of the hospital, such as the emergency department, where patients often feel forgotten, as the doctors are inundated attempting to see everyone. You can make a huge difference just by talking to them and letting them know that everything is moving forward, even if slowly.

2.4   CONCLUSION

Entering a clinical setting for the first time as an engineer can be an intimidating and daunting experience. Garnering valuable information and learning from the clinical experience can be an even more difficult endeavor. I hope that gaining a general understanding of hospital culture and protocol has made you feel more prepared to enter the hospital as an observing student.

CHAPTER 3

MEDICAL TERMINOLOGY

Ilhami Kovanlikaya and Yi Wang

Of all the novel aspects one experiences when working in a hospital for the first time – the protocol, the attitude, the attire, the professional structure and rules – the medical vocabulary may be the most difficult to grasp. The dialogue of health care professionals may be so foreign to a new student that it initially sounds like another language. This is because the vast amount of medical vocabulary and terms, most of which are not used in colloquial speech, are essentially another language in themselves. A student new to the hospital setting is not expected to be an expert in medical vocabulary. However, students can profoundly enrich their hospital experience by learning several essential medical roots, vocabulary words, and terms, allowing them to go from unengaged bystanders to knowledgeable and active participants who are able to follow the medical dialogue.

3.1   ANATOMICAL POSITION AND BODY PLANES

Anatomical Position. In order to standardize terminology regarding the human body and its movements, anatomists have created a universal "anatomical position". In this position, the body is assumed to be standing, with the feet together, the arms palm forward on the side with the thumbs facing away from the body.

Cartesian 3D coordinate system is then used to describe the human body in the anatomic position (Fig.3.1). The xyz axes are defined as right-left, anterior-posterior, and superior-inferior. Corresponding xy plane is defined as the transverse (horizontal) plane; yz plane as the sagittal (median) plane, and xz plane as the coronal (frontal) plane.

Additionally, to describe the distance relationship relative to the body center, proximal and distal modifiers are used. To describe the distance relationship relative to the midline (z-axis in Fig.3.1), medial and lateral modifiers are used.

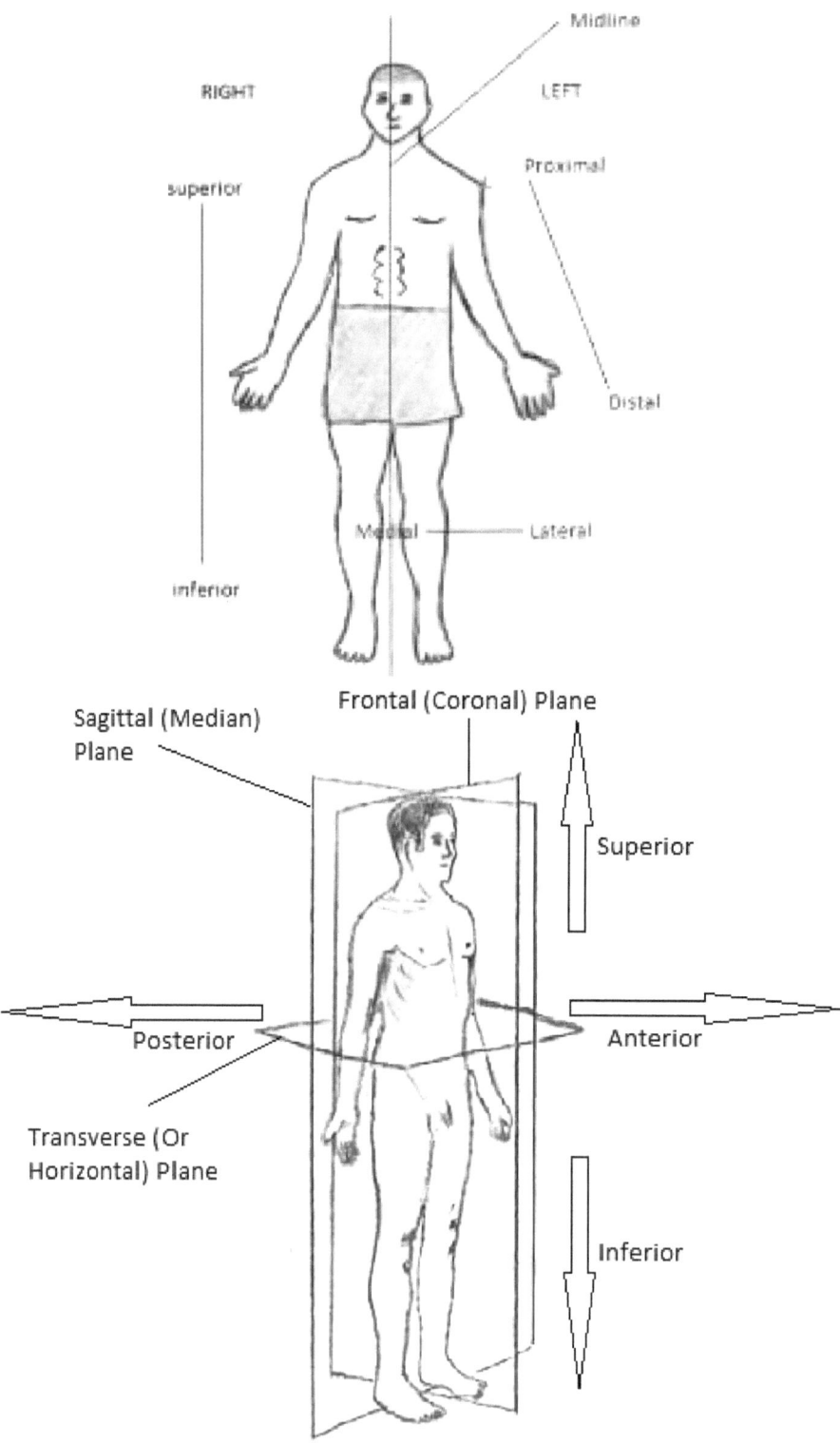

Fig.3.1. Anatomical position (top) and planes of the body (bottom).

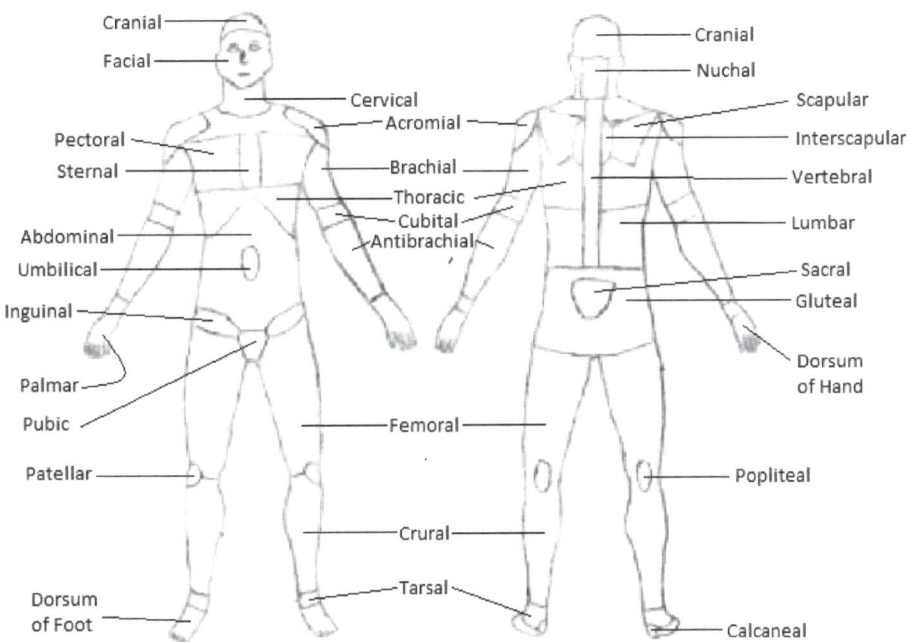

Fig.3.2. Terminology describing body parts.

The planes and directions of the coordinate system illustrated in Fig.3.1 are summarized as the following.

- Supine: Body is lying down on back with face up.
- Prone: Body is lying face down with back facing upwards.
- Mid-Sagittal or Median Plane: The body is divided into equal right and left halves by this plane.
- Sagittal plane: Any plane parallel to the median plane.
- Frontal (Coronal) Plane: Vertical plane at right angle to median plane which divides the body into its anterior and posterior parts.
- Transverse plane: Horizontal plane of the body perpendicular to both frontal and sagittal planes that separates the body into its top and bottom parts.
- Oblique plane: Any plane through the body that is not parallel to the other planes described above.
- Medial: Structures of the body are nearer the midline/towards midline.
- Lateral: Away from the middle of the body.
- Anterior: Towards the front of the body.
- Posterior: Towards the back of the body.
- Inferior: Towards the feet; lower.

- Superior: Towards the head; higher.
- Distal: Away from the origin; farther from the point of attachment.
- Proximal: Closer to the origin; closer to the point of attachment.

Major body parts are illustrated in Fig.3.2 and summarized in the following.
- Cranial: related to the head
- Cervical: related to the cervix or neck.
- Thoracic: related to the thoracic trunk.
- Abdominal: related to the abdomen.
- Pelvic: related to the pelvis.
- Dorsal: Towards the back of the body.
- Ventral: Towards the front of the body.
- Rostral: Towards the front of the head.
- Caudal: Towards the back; the tail.

3.2   MEDICAL TERMINOLOGY SYSTEM

Medical terminology can be systematically comprehended according root word, prefix and suffix. Determination of the root meaning will usually establish the main thrust of the term. Root words are commonly derived from Greek or Latin source language. Prefixes are used to indicate location, number and time, and suffixes to indicate condition and process. When a medical term involves two or more body parts, individual root words are joined using the letter "o", as in cardiothoracic. Challenges in mastering medical terms include both Greek and Latin root words for the same organ, root words usually do not stand alone as complete words, and plural forms are in the source language.

It may be useful for students to have a crash course of study or a quick review of the commonly used Greek/Latin root words, prefixes and suffixes. These terms can be organized into two categories, 1) anatomic and medical (Table 3.1), and 2) relational (Table 3.2). Accordingly, the following two tables list root words, prefixes and suffixes commonly used in medicine for engineering students to have a quick study and reference.

The root "keys" from Tables.3.1&2 can be practiced by reviewing the medical vocabulary list in the Appendix.

Table 3.1. Anatomic and medical root words, prefixes and suffixes.

ROOT, PRE/SUF-FIX	MEANING	EXAMPLE	EXPLANATION
Limb and skeletal			
arthr	joint	arthritis	joint inflammation
carpal	wrist	carpal tunnel syndrome	wrist nerve pain
chir	hand	chiropractic	(hand) manipulation of body structure
dactyl	finger	dactylography	fingerprint study
manus	hand	manubrium	hand like upper portion of sternum
my	muscle	myocardium	muscle in heart
oste	bone	osteoporosis	bone porous process
pedal	foot	pedestrian	walking people
pod	foot	podiatrist	foot doctor
tarsal	ankle	tarsal bones	bones in ankle
Head and neck			
audit	hear	auditory	of hearing
aur	ear	auriscope	device to look into the ear
bucc	cheek	buccopharyngeal fascia	cheek to pharynx connective tissue
caput	head	caput medusae	like medusa's head – enlarged paraumbilical vein
cereb	brain	Cerebrum	brain (upper part)
cervic	neck	Cervical	of neck
col(l)	neck	Collar	around neck
corona	crown	Coronary	like a crown
encephala	head	encephalitis	brain inflammation
hypno	sleep	Hypnosis	sleep like state
lingu	tongue	linguistics	tongue work (speech) study
nas	nosc	nasal	of nose
neuro	nerve	neurology	nerve system study
oculo	eye	ocular migraine	retinal disease accompanied by migraine headache
olfact	smell	olfactory	of smell

21

ophthalm	eye	ophthalmology	eye system and disease study
opia	vision	Myopia	squint eye – nearsighted
ot	ear	Otoscope	device to look into the ear
phasia	speech	dysphasia	malfunction/disorder in speech
psycho	mind	psychology	mind study
rhin	nose	Rhinoplasty	nose plastic surgery
somn	Sleep	Insomnia	inability to fall asleep
tact	touch	Tactile	relating to touch sense
Body			
angi	vessel	angiography	vessel imaging
cardi	heart	Cardiology	heart study
chol	bile	Cholera	bile (gastrointestinal) symptom
corp-	body	Corpus	body (dead) collection of writing
coxal	hip	Coxa	hip joint
cut	skin	Cutaneous	of skin
derm	skin	dermatology	skin study
diure	urinate	Diuretic	(increase) urination
emia	blood	Anemia	lacking blood
glute	buttock	Gluteal	relating to buttock
hem	blood	Hematoma	blood mass
hepat	liver	hepatitis	liver inflammation
hist	tissue	histology	tissue study
hyster	uterus	hysterectomy	uterus excision
inguinal	groin	inguinal ligament	in inguinal canal, connective the ilium to the public bone
lapar	abdomen	laparoscopy	abdomen exam
mamm	breast	mammography	breast imaging
mast	breast	mastectomy	breast excision
nephr	kidney	nephrology	kidney study
pneumon	Lung/air	pneumonia	lung inflammation
pulmo	lung	pulmonary	relating to lung
ren	kidney	renal artery	artery supplying kidney
soma	body	somatization	conversion from mental to body pain
some	body	lysosome	loosening body – membrane bound cell

			organelle
steth	chest	stethoscope	chest exam device (hearing chest sound)
thorac	chest	thoracic	of chest
vent	belly	ventral hernia	protrusion (through a wall/connective tissue) of belly
viscero	organ	viscerosomatic	relating to both internal organ and outer body trunk
Medicine			
alg	Pain	Neuralgia	pain caused by a nerve
brady	slow	bradycardia	slow beating heart (<50bpm)
dys	Improper, bad	dystrophy	abnormal growth
ectomy	excision/cut	endorectomy	cut from inside, as in carotid endorectomy
gangli	Swelling, mass	ganglion	cell cluster in peripheral nervous system
iatr	Medical care	Podiatry	feet medical care
itis, ia	inflammation	dermatitis	skin inflammation
mal	Bad	Malignant	"badly bear", causing harm
neo	new	neoplasm	new creation (abnormal growth) - tumor
oma	growth	carcinoma	cancer of epithelial cells: growing body looking like a crab
onc	tumor	oncogenic	relating to tumor formation
osis	process	narcosis	sleep/death process: cell injury of premature death
path	disease	pathology	disease study
peps, pept	Digestion	Peptic	aiding digestion
scopy	examination	thoracoscopy	thoracic cavity examination
septi	rotten	antiseptic	opposing decay
tachy	rapid	tachycardia	fast beating heart (>100bpm)
therap	treatment	therapeutic	of treatment of disease

thromb	clot	thrombosis	blood clotting process
trauma	wound	traumatic	wounded
tox	poison	toxicology	poison study
zyme	ferment	enzyme	biological catalyst

Table 3.2. Relational root words, prefixes and suffixes.

ROOT, PRE/SUF-FIX	MEANING	EXAMPLE	EXPLANATION
a	lacking	anemia	lacking blood
ab	away from	abduct	move away from the median plane
ac-, ad-	toward	accelerate, admittance	celer – fast mittere - send
ana	throughout	anatomy	through cut
ante	before	antebrachium	forearm
anti	against	antibiotics	against bacteria
apo	separation	apophysis	projecting part of an organ
bi	double	bicuspid	two cusps
cata	down	catabolism	breaking down molecules
cle, cula	diminutive	tubercle	small nodule
con, com	together	conjugate	link together
contra	opposite	contralateral	opposite side
de	reduce	debug	remove bugs
di	apart	dissect	cut apart piece by piece
dia	through	diagnosis	knowledge through (studying symptom)
e, ex, extra	away from	excision	cut from outside (cise=cut)
ecto	outside	ectoderm	outer germ layer
endo	inside	endocardium	inner layer of the heart
epi	upon, over	epidemic	upon people – spreading from person to person
fer, ferent	carry	afferent	carry toward
ger	old age	geriatrics	elderly medicine
graph	record	radiograph	x-ray image
gyn	female	genecology	female reproductive medicine
hyper	excessive	hyperextension	beyond normal

hypo	under	hypoglycemia	low sugar level in blood
in	in	incision	cut from inside
infra	beneath	infraorbital	below the orbit
inter	between	intervertebral	between vertebrae
intra	within	intravenous	inside vein
ipsi	same	ipsilateral	same side
ject	throw	ejection	throwing out
kine	motion	akinesia	slowness from impaired muscle
later	side	bilateral	two sides
leuk	white	leukemia	white blood cell increase
mes, medi, mid	middle	mesoderm	middle germ layer
meta	after	metacarpal	after the wrist
necr	dead	necrology	list of people died recently
oid	resembling	xiphoid	shaped like a sword
-ole,-olus	diminutive	malleolus	little hammer
ortho	straight	orthodontist	straightening teeth dentist
pan	all	panacea	a cure for all diseases
peri	around	periodontal	around tooth
plas/t/m	form	cytoplasm	cell substance
post	after	postnatal	after birth
pre	before	prenephron	before the final kidney
retro	behind	retrosternal	behind the sternum
rhod	red	rhodopsin	purple pigment in the retina
rrhea/age	discharge	hemorrhage	blood discharge
sclero	hard	arteriosclerosis	hardening of the arterial walls
se	apart	serum	liquid separated from blood
sub	beneath	subclavian	beneath the clavicle
super	above	suprasternal	above the sternum
trans	through	transurethral	through urethra

Glossary. Basic medical terms.

A

abdomen: The part of the body between the diaphragm and pelvis containing the digestive organs.

abduction: The movement of a body part away from the axis or midline of the body.

absorption: The transport of molecules across epithelial membranes into the body fluids

acidosis: An increased acidity in the blood and other body tissue (i.e., an increased hydrogen ion concentration) that lowers the arterial pH to below 7.35.

acromegaly: The hypersecretion of growth hormone from the pituitary gland after maturity which causes enlargement of the extremities, such as the nose, jaws, fingers, and toes.

active transport: The movement of molecules or ions across a cell membrane in a direction against their concentration gradient. An expenditure of cellular energy (ATP) is required.

active immunity: Immunity involving sensitization, in which antibody production is stimulated by prior exposure to an antigen.

adduction: The movement of a body part toward the axis or midline of the body.

adenohypophysis: The anterior, glandular lobe of the pituitary.

adenoids: The tonsils; located in the nasopharynx.

adrenergic: A term used to describe the actions of epinephrine, norepinephrine, or other molecules with similar activity.

adventitia (serosa): The outermost epithelial layer of a visceral organ.

afferent: Bringing to or leading towards an organ or part (opposed to efferent).

alimentary canal (gastrointestinal tract): The tubular portion of the digestive tract.

allergy: A state of hypersensitivity caused by exposure to allergens. It results in the liberation of histamine and other molecules with histamine like effects.

alveolus: An individual air capsule within the lung which is the basic functional unit of respiration. The socket that secures a tooth (tooth socket).

ampulla: A saclike enlargement of a duct or tube.

anaphylaxis: A severe allergic reaction that can result in cardiovascular shock and death.

anastomosis: An interconnecting of blood vessels or nerves that form a network plexus.

anatomical position: An erect body stance with the feet together, the arms palm forward on the side with the thumbs facing away from the body.

anatomy: The branch of science concerned with the structure of the body and the relationship of its organs.

androgens: Steroids containing 18 carbons that have masculinizing effects; primarily those hormones (such as testosterone) secreted by the testes.

anemia: An abnormal reduction in the red blood cell count, hemoglobin concentration, or hematocrit, or any combination of these measurements.

angina pectoris: A thoracic pain, often referred to the left pectoral and arm area, caused by myocardial ischemia

anterior (ventral): Toward the front; the opposite of posterior, or dorsal.

anterior pituitary: Adenohypophysis.

antibody: An Immunoglobin (Ig), a specialized protein secreted by B lymphocytes which is responsible for humoral immunity.

antigen: A molecule that can induce the production of antibodies and react in a specific manner with antibodies.

anus: The terminal opening of the GI tract.

aorta: The major systemic vessel of the arterial system of the body, emerging from the left ventricle.

apex: The tip or pointed end of a conical structure.

aphasia: Defects in speech, writing, or in the comprehension of spoken or written language caused by brain damage or disease.

appendix: A short pouch that attaches to the cecum that is a part of a large bowel.

arachnoid mater: The web-like middle covering (meninx) of the central nervous system.

arteriole: The smallest branches of an artery that lead to a capillary.

arteriosclerosis: Any one of a group of diseases characterized by thickening and hardening of the artery wall and the narrowing of its lumen.

arteriovenous anastomoses: Direct connections between arteries and veins that bypass capillary beds.

artery: A blood vessel that carries blood away from the heart.

atherosclerosis: A common type of arteriosclerosis found in medium and larger arteries in which raised areas within the tunica intima are formed from smooth muscle cells, cholesterol, and other lipids. These plaques occlude arteries and serve as sites for the formation of thrombi.

atrium: Either of the two superior chambers of the heart that receive venous blood.

atrophy: A gradual wasting away or decrease in the size of a tissue or an organ.

auditory: Pertaining to the structures of the ear associated with hearing.

autonomic nervous system (ANS): The sympathetic and parasympathetic portions of the nervous system that function to control the actions of the visceral organs and skin.

axilla: The depressed hollow commonly called the armpit.

axon: The elongated process of a nerve cell that transmits an impulse away from the cell body of a neuron.

B

basal metabolic rate (BMR): The rate of metabolism (expressed as oxygen consumption or heat production) under resting or basal conditions.

basal nucleus (basal ganglion): A mass of nerve cell bodies located deep within a cerebral hemisphere.

benign: Not a threat to life or long-term health, not malignant.

bifurcate : Forked; divided into two branches.

bile: A liver secretion that is stored and concentrated in the gallbladder and released through the common bile duct into the duodenum. It is essential for the absorption of fats.

bilirubin: Bile pigment derived from the breakdown of the heme portion of hemoglobin.

blood-brain barrier (BBB): A specialized mechanism that inhibits the passage of certain materials from the blood into brain tissue and cerebrospinal fluid.

brachial plexus: A network of nerve fibers that arise from spinal nerves C5-C8 and T1 which supply the upper extremities.

bradycardia: A slow cardiac rate; fewer than 60 beats per minute.

brain stem: The portion of the brain consisting of the medulla oblongata, pons, and midbrain.

bronchus: A branch of the trachea that leads to a lung.

C

cancer: A tumor characterized by abnormally rapid cell division and the loss of specialized tissue characteristics, usually refers to malignant tumors.

capillary: A microscopic blood vessel that connects an arteriole and a venule; the functional unit of the circulatory system.

cardiac output: The volume of blood pumped per minute by either the right or left ventricle.

cardiogenic shock: Shock that results from low cardiac output in heart disease.

catabolism: The metabolic breakdown of complex molecules into simpler ones, often resulting in a release of energy.

catecholamines: A group of molecules including epinephrine, norepinephrine, L-dopa, and related molecules with effects similar to those produced by activation of the sympathetic nervous system.

cauda equine: The lower end of the spinal cord where the roots of spinal nerves have a tail-like appearance.

cell: The structural and functional unit of an organism; the smallest structure capable of performing all the functions necessary for life.

cell-mediated immunity: Immunological defense provided by T cell lymphocytes that come within close proximity of their victim cells (as opposed to humoral immunity provided by the secretion of antibodies by plasma cells).

central nervous system (CNS): Part of the nervous system consisting of the brain and the spinal cord.

cerebellum: The portion of the brain concerned with the coordination of skeletal muscle contraction.

cerebrospinal fluid (CSF): A fluid produced by the choroid plexus in the ventricles of the brain. It fills the ventricles and surrounds the central nervous system in association with the meninges.

cerebrum: The largest portion of the brain, composed of the right and left hemispheres.

cervical: Pertaining to the neck or a necklike portion of an organ.

cervix: The narrow necklike portion of an organ.

chemotaxis: The movement of an organism or a cell, such as a leukocyte, toward a chemical stimulus.

chiasma: A crossing of nerve tracts from one side of the CNS to the other.

cholesterol: A 27-carbon steroid that serves as the precursor of steroid hormones.

cholinergic: Denoting nerve endings that liberate acetylcholine as a neurotransmitter, such as those of the parasympathetic system.

choroid plexus: A mass of vascular capillaries from which cerebrospinal fluid is secreted into the ventricles of the brain.

chromosomes: Structures in the nucleus that contain the genes for genetic expression.

cilia: Microscopic hairlike processes that move in a wavelike manner on the exposed surfaces of certain epithelial cells.

circadian rhythms: Physiological changes that repeat at about 24-hour intervals. These are often synchronized with changes in the external environment, such as the day-night cycles.

circle of Willis (cerebral arterial circle): an arterial polygon as the internal carotid and vertebral systems anastomose around the optic chiasm and infundibulum of the pituitary stalk.

cirrhosis: Liver disease characterized by loss of normal microscopic structure, which is replaced by fibrosis and nodular regeneration.

collateral: A small side branch of a blood vessel or nerve fiber.

colon : Large intestine.

congenital: Present at the time of birth.

congestive heart failure: The heart fails to pump blood at a rate commensurate with the requirements of the metabolizing tissues as a result of heart disease or hypertension. This condition is associated with breathlessness, excessive tiredness and edema.

connective tissue: It is a binding and supportive tissue with abundant matrix.

contralateral: Taking place or originating in a corresponding part on the opposite side of the body.

conus medullaris: The inferior, tapering portion of the spinal cord.

cornea: The transparent, convex, anterior portion of the outer layer of the eyeball.

coronal plane (frontal plane): A vertical plane that divides the body into anterior (ventral) and posterior (dorsal) portions.

coronary circulation: The arterial and venous blood circulation to the wall of the heart.

corpus callosum: A large tract of white matter within the brain that connects the right and left cerebral hemispheres.

cortex: 1.The outer layer of an internal organ or body structure, as of the kidney or adrenal gland. 2. The convoluted layer of gray matter that covers the surface of each cerebral hemisphere.

corticosteroids: Steroid hormones of the adrenal cortex, consisting of glucocorticoids (such as hydrocortisone) and mineralocorticoids (such as aldosterone).

cranial: Pertaining to the cranium.

cranial nerves: One of 12 pairs of nerves that arise from the brain.

cranium: The bones of the skull that enclose or support the brain and the organs of sight, hearing, and balance.

Cushing's syndrome: Symptoms caused by the hypersecretion of adrenal steroid hormones as a result of tumors of the adrenal cortex or ACTH secreting tumors of the anterior pituitary.

cyanosis: A bluish discoloration of the skin or mucous membranes due to insufficient oxygen in the blood.

cytology: The science dealing with the study of cells.

cytoplasm: In a cell, the cell substance between the cell membrane and the nucleus, containing the cytosol, organelles, cytoskeleton, and various particles.

D

decussation: A crossing of nerve fibers from one side of the CNS to the other.

defecation: The elimination of feces from the rectum through the anal canal and out the anus.

dendrite: A nerve cell short process that transmits impulses toward a neuron cell body.

dermis: The second, or deep, layer of skin beneath the epidermis.

diabetes insipidus: A condition in which inadequate amounts of antidiuretic hormone (ADH) are secreted by the posterior pituitary. It results in the inadequate reabsorption of water by the kidney tubules; thus, in the excretion of a large volume of dilute urine.

diabetes mellitus: The appearance of glucose in the urine due to the presence of high plasma glucose concentrations, even in the fasting state. This disease is caused by either lack of sufficient insulin secretion or inadequate responsiveness of the target tissues to the effects of insulin.

diaphragm: A sheetlike dome of muscle and connective tissue that separates the thoracic and abdominal cavities.

diaphysis: The shaft of a long bone.

diarrhea: Abnormal frequency of defecation accompanied by abnormal liquidity of the feces.

diastole: The sequence of the cardiac cycle during which a heart chamber wall is relaxed.

diencephalon: A major region of the brain that includes the third ventricle, thalamus, hypothalamus, and pituitary gland.

digestion: The process by which larger molecules of food substance are broken down mechanically and chemically into smaller molecules that can be absorbed.

distal: Away from the midline or origin; the opposite of proximal.

diuretic: An agent that promotes the excretion of urine, thereby lowering blood volume and pressure.

DNA (Deoxyribonucleic acid): composed of nucleotide bases and deoxyribose sugar. It is found in all living cells and contains the genetic code.

dorsal: Pertaining to the back or posterior portion of a body part; the opposite of ventral; also called posterior.

dorsiflexion: Movement at the ankle as the dorsum of the foot is elevated.

duodenum: The first portion of the small intestine that leads from the pylorus of the stomach to the jejunum.

dura mater: The outermost meninx covers the central nervous system.

dyspnea: Difficulty in breathing.

E

ECG: Electrocardiogram.

edema: An excessive accumulation of fluid in the body tissues.

efferent: Conveying away from the center of an organ or structure.

efferent neuron: Motor neuron.

electrocardiogram: A recording of the electrical activity that accompanies the cardiac cycle; ECG or EKG.

electroencephalogram (EEG): A recording of the brainwave patterns or electrical impulses of the brain from electrodes placed on the scalp.

electromyogram: A recording of the electrical impulses or activity of skeletal muscles using surface electrodes; EMG.

embryology: The study of prenatal development from conception through the eighth week in utero.

emphysema: A lung disease in which the alveoli are destroyed and the remaining alveoli become larger. It results in decreased vital capacity and increased airway resistance.

endocardium: The endothelial lining of the heart chambers and valves.

endocrine gland: A ductless, hormone-producing gland that is part of the endocrine system.

endogenous: Denoting a product or process arising from within the body (as opposed to exogenous products or influences from external sources).

endorphins: A group of endogenous opiate molecules that may act as a natural analgesic.

endothelium: The layer of epithelial tissue that forms the thin inner lining of blood vessels and heart chambers.

enteric: The term referring to the small intestine.

enzyme: A protein catalyst that increases the rate of specific chemical reactions.

eosinophil: A type of white blood cell characterized by the presence of cytoplasmic granules that become stained by acidic eosin dye.

epidermis: The outermost layer of the skin, composed of several stratified squamous epithelial layers.

epidural space: A space between the spinal dura mater and the bone of the vertebral canal.

epiphysis: The end segment of a long bone, separated from the diaphysis early in life by an epiphyseal plate but later becoming part of the larger bone.

epithelial tissue: One of the four basic tissue types; the type of tissue that covers or lines all exposed body surfaces

erythrocyte: A red blood cell.

esophagus: A tubular portion of the GI tract that leads from the pharynx to the stomach as it passes through the thoracic cavity.

essential amino acids: Those eight amino acids in adults or nine amino acids in children that cannot be made by the human body; therefore, they must be obtained in the diet.

estrogens: Any of several female sex hormones secreted from the ovarian (graafian) follicle.

etiology: The study of cause, especially of disease, including the origin and what pathogens, if any, are involved.

eustachian canal: Auditory tube.

exocrine gland: A gland that secretes its product to an epithelial surface, directly or through ducts.

expiration: The process of expelling air from the lungs through breathing out; also called exhalation.

extension: A movement that increases the angle between parts of a joint.

external: Located on or toward the surface.

extrinsic: Pertaining to an outside or external origin.

F

falx cerebri: A fold of dura mater which extends between the right and left cerebral hemispheres.

fascia: A tough sheet of fibrous tissue binding the skin to underlying muscles or supporting and separating muscles.

fasciculus: A small bundle of muscle or nerve fibers.

feces (gaita): Material expelled from the large bowel during defecation, composed of undigested food residue, bacteria, and secretions; also called stool.

fertilization: The fusion of an ovum and spermatozoon.

fetus: An unborn human after 8 weeks of development.

fibrillation: A condition of rapid, irregular, and uncoordinated contraction of muscle fibers. If it occurs in the ventricles of the heart resulting in the inability of the myocardium to contract as a unit and pump blood, it can be fatal.

fibrin: The insoluble protein formed from fibrinogen by the enzymatic action of thrombin during the process of blood clot formation.

filum terminale: A fibrous, threadlike continuation of the pia mater, extending inferiorly from the terminal end of the spinal cord to the coccyx.

fissure: A groove or narrow cleft that separates two parts, such as the cerebral hemispheres of the brain.

flexion: A movement that decreases the angle between parts of a joint.

foramen, pl. foramina: An opening in an anatomical structure, usually in a bone, for the passage of a blood vessel or a nerve.

fossa: A depressed area, usually on a bone.

fourth ventricle: A cavity filled with cerebrospinal fluid which is located in the brain stem between the cerebellum and the medulla oblongata and the pons.

frontal: 1.the bone of the skull forming forehead. 2. A plane through the body, dividing the body into anterior and posterior portions; also called the coronal plane.

G

gallbladder: A pouchlike organ attached to the underside of the liver in which bile secreted by the liver is stored and concentrated.

ganglion: An aggregation of nerve cell bodies occurring outside the central nervous system.

gastrointestinal tract (GI tract): The portion of the digestive tract that includes the stomach, the small and large intestines.

gigantism: Abnormal body growth as a result of the excessive secretion of growth hormone.

gland: An organ that produces a specific substance or secretion.

glomerular filtration rate (GFR): The volume of filtrate produced per minute by both kidneys.

glomerulonephritis: Inflammation of the renal glomeruli, associated with fluid retention, edema, hypertension, and the appearance of protein in the urine.

glomerulus: A coiled tuft of capillaries surrounded by the glomerular capsule that filtrates urine from the blood.

glucocorticoid (corticosteroid): A steroid hormone secreted by the adrenal cortex which affects the metabolism of carbohydrates and to a lesser extend proteins and fats. It also has anti-inflammatory and immunosuppressive effects. Hydrocortisone (cortisol) is the major glucocorticoid in humans.

glycolysis: A complex biological process that occurs to convert glucose into pyruvic acid in order to provide energy for each living cell.

glycosuria: The excretion of an abnormal amount of glucose in the urine.

gonad: A reproductive organ, testis or ovary, that produces gametes and sex hormones.

gray matter: The major component of the central nervous system composed of nerve cell bodies and their dendrites (mostly unmyelinated nerve tissue).

growth hormone: A hormone secreted by the anterior pituitary that stimulates growth of the body that influences the metabolism of protein, carbohydrate, and fat throughout life.

gyrus: A convoluted elevation or ridge.

H

hay fever: A seasonal type of allergic rhinitis caused by pollen; it is characterized by itching and tearing of the eyes, swelling of the nasal mucosa, attacks of sneezing, and asthma.

heart murmur: An extra or unusual auscultatory sound heard during a heartbeat as a result of structural defects of the valves or septum.

hematocrit: The ratio of packed red blood cells to total blood volume in a centrifuged sample of blood, expressed as a percentage.

heme: The iron-containing red pigment that, together with the protein globin, forms hemoglobin.

hemoglobin: The iron-containing oxygen-transport metalloprotein in the red blood cells that transports oxygen.

hemopoiesis (hematopoiesis): The production of red blood cells.

heparin: A mucopolysaccharide that prevents clots in the blood vessels.

hepatitis: Inflammation of the liver.

hiatus: An opening or fissure; a foramen.

high-density lipoproteins (HDLs): The carrier protein for lipids, such as cholesterol, that appear to offer some protection from atherosclerosis.

hilum (hilus): A concave or depressed area where vessels or nerves enter or exit an organ.

histamine: A compound that stimulates vasodilation and increases capillary permeability. It is responsible for many of the symptoms of inflammation and allergy.

histology: Microscopic anatomy of the structure and function of tissues.

homeostasis: The dynamic constancy of the internal environment, the maintenance of which is the principal function of physiological regulatory mechanisms.

horizontal (transverse) plane: A directional plane that divides the body, organ, or appendage into superior and inferior or proximal and distal portions.

hormone: A chemical substance produced in an endocrine gland and secreted into the bloodstream to cause an effect in a specific target organ.

humoral immunity (antibody-mediated immunity): The form of acquired immunity in which antibody molecules are secreted in response to antigenic stimulation (as opposed to cell mediated immunity).

hyaline membrane disease (respiratory distress syndrome): A disease affecting premature infants who lack pulmonary surfactant. It is characterized by collapse of the alveoli (atelectasis) and pulmonary edema.

hydrocortisone (cortisol): The principal corticosteroid hormone secreted by the adrenal cortex, with glucocorticoid action.

hydrophilic: Having an affinity for water.

hydrophobic: Denoting a substance that repels and that is repelled by water.

hypercapnia: Excessive concentration of carbon dioxide in the blood.

hyperglycemia: An abnormally increased concentration of glucose in the blood.

hyperplasia: An increase in organ size due to an increase in cell numbers as a result of mitotic cell division (in contrast to hypertrophy).

hypersensitivity: abnormal immune response that may be immediate (due to antibodies of the IgE class) or delayed (due to cell-mediated immunity).

hypertension: Elevated or excessive blood pressure.

hypertonic: Denoting a solution with a greater solute concentration and thus a greater osmotic pressure than plasma.

hypertrophy: Growth of an organ due to an increase in the size of its cells (in contrast to hyperplasia).

hyperventilation: A high rate and depth of breathing that results in a decrease in the blood carbon dioxide concentration to below normal.

hypothalamus: A portion of the forebrain within the diencephalon that lies below the thalamus, where it functions as an autonomic nerve center and regulates the pituitary gland.

hypovolemic shock: A rapid fall in blood pressure as a result of diminished blood volume.

hypoxemia: A low oxygen concentration of the arterial blood.

I

immunization: The process of increasing one's resistance to pathogens.

immunoglobulins: Subclasses of the gamma globulin fraction of plasma proteins that have antibody functions, providing humoral immunity.

inferior vena cava: A large systemic vein that collects blood from the body regions inferior to the level of the heart and returns it to the right atrium.

inguinal: Pertaining to the groin region.

inspiration: The act of breathing air into the alveoli of the lungs; also called inhalation.

insulin: A polypeptide hormone secreted by the beta cells of the pancreatic islets that promotes the cellular uptake of blood glucose and, therefore, lowers the blood glucose concentration. Insulin deficiency results in hyperglycemia and diabetes mellitus (type 2 diabetes). A condition in which the pancreas produces little or no insulin results in type 1 diabetes.

interferons: A group of small proteins that inhibit the multiplication of viruses inside host cells and that also have antitumor properties.

internal: Toward the center, away from the surface of the body.

intervertebral disc: A pad of fibrocartilage located between the bodies of adjacent vertebrae.

intrinsic: Situated within or pertaining to internal origin.

in vitro: Occurring outside the body, in a test tube or other artificial environment.

in vivo: Occurring within the body.

ipsilateral: On the same side (as opposed to contralateral).

ischemia: A rate of blood flow to an organ that is inadequate to supply sufficient oxygen and maintain aerobic respiration in that organ.

isthmus: A narrow neck or portion of tissue connecting two structures.

J

jaundice: A condition characterized by high blood bilirubin levels and staining of the tissues with bilirubin, which imparts a yellow color to the skin and mucous membranes.

jejunum: The middle portion of the small intestine, located between the duodenum and the ileum.

K

ketoacidosis: A type of metabolic acidosis resulting from the excessive production of ketone bodies, as in diabetes mellitus.

Krebs cycle: A cyclic metabolic pathway in the matrix of mitochondria by which the acetic acid part of acetyl coenzyme (CoA) is oxidized and substrates are provided for reactions that are coupled to the formation of adenosine triphosphate (ATP).

L

lacrimal gland: A tear-secreting gland, located on the superior lateral portion of the eyeball underneath the upper eyelid.

lactation: The production and secretion of milk by the mammary glands.

large intestine: The last major portion of the GI tract, consisting of the cecum, colon, rectum, and anal canal.

larynx: The structure located between the pharynx and trachea that houses the vocal cords; commonly called the voice box.

lateral: Pertaining to the side; farther from the midplane.

lateral ventricle: A cavity within the cerebral hemisphere of the brain that is filled with cerebrospinal fluid.

lesion: A wounded or damaged area.

leukocyte: A white blood cell.

ligament: A tough cord or fibrous band of connective tissue that binds bone to bone to strengthen and provide flexibility to a joint. It also may support viscera.

low-density lipoproteins (LDLs): Plasma proteins that transport triglycerides and cholesterol. They are believed to contribute to arteriosclerosis.

lower extremity A lower appendage, including the hip, thigh, knee, leg, and foot.

lumbar: Pertaining to the region of the loins.

lumen: The space within a tubular structure through which a substance passes.

lymph: A clear, plasma like fluid that flows through lymphatic vessels.

lymphatic system: The lymphatic vessels and lymph nodes.

lymphocyte: A type of white blood cell which usually constitutes about 20% to 25% of the white blood cell count.

M

macrophage: A wandering phagocytic cell.

malignant: Threatening to life; virulent. Of a tumor, cancerous, tending to metastasize.

matrix: The intercellular substance of a tissue.

meatus: A passageway or opening into a structure.

medial: Toward or closer to the midplane of the body.

mediastinum: The partition in the center of the thorax between the two pleural cavities. The heart is situated within.

medulla: The center portion of an organ.

medulla oblongata: A portion of the brain stem located between the spinal cord and the pons.

meninges: A group of three fibrous membranes covering the central nervous system, composed of the dura mater, arachnoid mater, and pia mater.

mesencephalon: The midbrain, which contains the corpora quadrigemina and the cerebral peduncles.

metabolism: The sum total of the chemical changes that occur within a cell.

arteriole: Passes through a capillary network and empties into a venule.

metastasis: The spread of a disease from one organ or body part to another.

midsagittal: A plane that divides the body into equal right and left halves; also called the median plane or midplane.

mitosis: The process of cell division that results in two identical daughter cells containing the same number of chromosomes.

mitral valve: The left atrioventricular heart valve; also called the bicuspid valve.

mucosa: A mucous membrane that lines cavities and tracts the opening to the exterior.

myelin sheath: A sheath surrounding axons formed by successive wrappings of a neuroglial cell membrane.

myocardium: The cardiac muscle layer of the heart.

N

nasopharynx: The first or uppermost chamber of the pharynx, positioned posterior to the nasal cavity and extending down to the soft palate.

necrosis: Cellular death or tissue death due to disease or trauma.

neonatal: The stage of life from birth to the end of 4 weeks.

neoplasm: A new, abnormal growth of tissue, as in a tumor.

nerve: A bundle of nerve fibers outside the central nervous system.

neuron: The structural and functional unit of the nervous system, composed of a cell body, dendrites, and an axon; also called a nerve cell.

nucleus: A spheroid body within a cell that contains the genetic factors of the cell.

nystagmus: Involuntary oscillary movements of the eye.

O

olfactory: Pertaining to the sense of smell.

oncotic pressure: The colloid osmotic pressure of solutions produced by proteins. In plasma, it serves to counterbalance the outward filtration of fluid from capillaries due to hydrostatic pressure.

optic: Pertaining to the eye.

orifice: An opening into a body cavity or tube.

osseous tissue: Bone tissue.

osteomalacia: Softening of bones due to a deficiency of vitamin D and calcium.

osteoporosis: Demineralization of bone, seen most commonly in postmenopausal women and patients who are inactive or paralyzed.

ovary: The female gonad in which ova and certain sexual hormones are produced.

P

palmar: Pertaining to the palm of the hand.

palpation: Examining the body by touching and feeling.

papillae: Small, nipple like projections.

paranasal sinus: An air chamber lined with a mucous membrane that communicates with the nasal cavity.

parathyroids: Small endocrine glands embedded on the posterior surface of the thyroid glands that are concerned with calcium metabolism.

parietal: Pertaining to a wall of an organ or cavity.

parotid gland: One of the paired salivary glands located on the side of the face over the masseter muscle just anterior to the ear and connected to the oral cavity through a salivary duct.

pathogen: Any disease-producing microorganism or substance.

pelvis: A basin like bony structure formed by the sacrum and ossa coxae.

pericardium: A protective serous membrane that surrounds the heart.

periosteum: A fibrous connective tissue covering the outer surface of bone.

peripheral nervous system: The nerves and ganglia of the nervous system that lie outside of the brain and spinal cord; PNS.

peristalsis: Rhythmic contractions of smooth muscle in the walls of various tubular organs by which the contents are forced onward.

peritoneum: The serous membrane that lines the abdominal cavity and covers the abdominal visceral organs.

phalanx (pl. phalanges): A bone of a finger or toe.

pharynx: The organ of the digestive system and respiratory system located at the back of the oral and nasal cavities that extends to the larynx anteriorly and to the esophagus posteriorly; also called the throat.

pineal gland: A small cone-shaped gland located in the roof of the third ventricle.

pituitary gland: A small, pea-shaped endocrine gland situated on the interior surface of the diencephalonic region of the brain consisting of anterior and posterior lobes; also called the hypophysis.

plantar: Pertaining to the sole of the foot.

plasma: The fluid, extracellular portion of circulating blood.

plasma cells: Cells derived from B lymphocytes that produce and secrete large amounts of antibodies. They are responsible for humoral immunity.

platelets: Small fragments of specific bone marrow cells that function in blood coagulation; also called thrombocytes.

plexus: A network of interlaced nerves or vessels.

polyuria: Excretion of an excessively large volume of urine in a given period.

pons: The portion of the brain stem just above the medulla oblongata and anterior to the cerebellum.

posterior: Toward the back; also called dorsal.

prone: Lying face-down.

proximal: Closer to the midplane of the body or to the origin of an appendage; the opposite of distal.

pulmonary: Pertaining to the lungs.

pyrogen: A fever-producing substance.

R

radionuclide scanning: A procedure using an IV radioactive substance that generates a color video image, with areas of intense color representing high tissue activity and areas of less intense color representing low tissue activity; used to study the activity of a tissue or organ (brain, heart, lungs, liver).

ramus: A branch of a bone, artery, or nerve.

renal: Pertaining to the kidney.

respiration: The exchange of gases between the external environment and the cells of an organism.

retina: The principal portion of the internal tunic of the eyeball that contains the photoreceptors.

rotation: The movement of a bone around its own longitudinal axis.

S

sagittal plane: A vertical plane, running parallel to the midsagittal plane, that divides the body into unequal right and left portions.

salivary gland: An accessory digestive gland that secretes saliva into the oral cavity.

septum: A membranous or fleshy wall dividing two cavities.

serum: Blood plasma with the clotting elements removed.

shock: As it relates to the cardiovascular system, this term refers to a rapid, uncontrolled fall in blood pressure, which in some cases becomes irreversible and leads to death.

sinus: A cavity or hollow space within a body organ, such as a bone.

somatic: Pertaining to the nonvisceral parts of the body.

spinal cord: The portion of the central nervous system that extends downward from the brain stem through the vertebral canal.

squamous: Flat or scalelike.

steroid: A lipid, derived from cholesterol, that has three 6-sided carbon rings and one 5-sided carbon ring. These form the steroid hormones of the adrenal cortex and gonads.

Stratified: Arranged in layers, or strata.

subarachnoid space: The space within the meninges, between the arachnoid mater and pia mater, where cerebrospinal fluid flows.

sulcus: A shallow impression or groove.

superficial; Toward or near the surface.

superior: Toward the upper part of a structure or toward the head; also called cephalic.

superior vena cava: A large systemic vein that collects blood from regions of the body superior to the heart and returns it to the right atrium.

systemic: Relating to the entire organism rather than to individual parts.

T

tachycardia: An excessively rapid heart rate, usually in excess of 100 beats per minute (in contrast to bradycardia, in which the heart rate is very slow).

tactile: Pertaining to the sense of touch.

tendon: A band of dense regular connective tissue that attaches muscle to bone.

thorax: The chest.

thrombocyte: A blood platelet.

thrombus: A blood clot produced by the formation of fibrin threads around a platelet plug.

trachea: The airway leading from the larynx to the bronchi composed of cartilaginous rings and a ciliated mucosal lining of the lumen; commonly called the windpipe.

transverse plane: A plane that divides the body into superior and inferior portions; also called a horizontal, or cross-sectional, plane.

trunk: The thorax and abdomen.

U

urea: The chief nitrogenous waste product of protein catabolism in the urine; formed in the liver from amino acids.

ureter: A tube that transports urine from the kidney to the urinary bladder.

urethra: A tube that transports urine from the urinary bladder to the outside of the body.

uterus: A hollow, muscular organ in which a fetus develops. It is located within the female pelvis between the urinary bladder and the rectum; commonly called the womb.

V

vacuole: A small space or cavity within the cytoplasm of a cell.

vasoconstriction: Narrowing of the lumen of blood vessels due to contraction of the smooth muscles in their walls.

vasodilation: Widening of the lumen of blood vessels due to relaxation of the smooth muscles in their walls.

vein: A blood vessel that conveys blood toward the heart.

vena cava: One of two large vessels that return deoxygenated blood to the right atrium of the heart.

ventilation: Breathing; the process of moving air into and out of the lungs.

ventral: Toward the front or facing surface; the opposite of dorsal.

ventricle: A cavity within an organ; especially those cavities in the brain that contain cerebrospinal fluid and those in the heart that contain blood to be pumped from the heart.

venule: A small vessel that carries venous blood from capillaries to a vein.

vertebral canal: The tube-like cavity extending through the vertebral column that contains the spinal cord; also called the spinal canal.

virulent: Pathogenic; able to cause disease.

viscera: The organs within the abdominal or thoracic cavities.

W

white matter: Bundles of myelinated axons located in the central nervous system.

Z

zygote: A fertilized egg cell formed by the union of a sperm cell and an ovum.

CHAPTER 4

MEDICAL IMAGING TECHNIQUES

Yi Wang, PhD

Medical Imaging has become an integral part of all facets of medicine, including radiological diagnosis, imaging guided intervention, and pathology. According to a recent poll about the most significant recent medical innovations, three of the top five medical innovations in the past 50 years are in imaging based diagnosis (MRI and CT Scanning and mammography) or imaging guided therapy (balloon angioplasty). Imaging is used to visualize tumors, guide surgical procedures, and identify pathologies; Imaging has been and will continue to be an essential component in the healthcare of many patients.

There are many imaging devices used in various ways in patient care. This chapter tries to explain the basic concepts of major imaging techniques currently used in hospitals. Fundamentally, medical imaging requires an energy to penetrate into the body to obtain information about tissue. A tissue sample may be obtained using a knife or a drill, which is called biopsy, and then be analyzed with various biochemical staining, which is called histology or pathology. In the following, we should focus on noninvasive methods using electromagnetic waves (x-ray at very high frequency, and magnetic resonance at radiofrequency), as well as ultrasound, that can penetrate the body with no or little harm.

4.1   X-RAY IMAGING – PROJECTION RADIOGRAPHY

Discovery of x-ray – one man's noise another man's signal. A partial-vacuum electrical discharge tube called a Crookes tube (named after one of its inventors William Crookes), which generates green fluorescence, had become widely available for physics research and entertainment after the 1870's. At that time, it was not known how the Crookes tube worked. Scientific investigations on the Crookes tube lead to two great discoveries in modern physics: the x-ray in 1895 by Wilhelm Roentgen and the electron in 1897 by JJ Thomson. With the development of quantum physics in the early part of the 20th century, we learned about the workings of the Crookes tube and x-ray generation. With a high voltage (>5kV) discharge, electrons are accelerated in the strong electric field to very high speed. As high-speed electrons pass near nuclei (bremsstrahlung) or knock out inner electrons (excited-ground state transition) in atoms in the anode, the glass tube, and air in the tube, x-rays are generated. X-rays had always been there in the Crookes tube. Indeed, early investigators including Ivan Puluj and Philipp von Lenard had noticed foggy marks on photographic plates nearby the Crookes tube in their experiments.

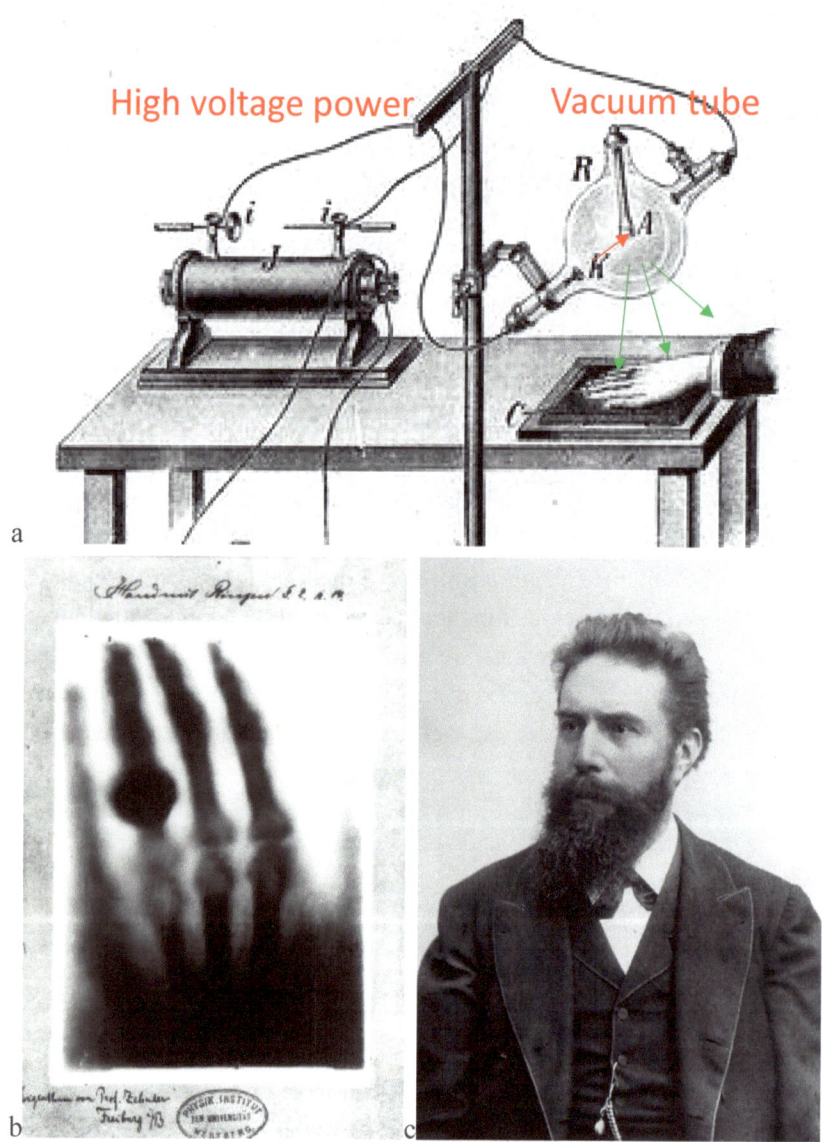

Fig.4.1. a) an early experimental setup for x-ray generation and imaging the hand, similar to that was used to produce the x-ray image of human body (b, the x-ray image of a hand of Roentgen's wife) by Roentgen (c).

On Friday November 8, 1895, Roentgen observed the same faint mark on the detector photo plate when the Crookes tube was covered with a black cardboard. He wanted to make sure the "faint marks" were there not as noise or error but as signal – an exciting new ray (x as the standard notation for unknown in mathematics, hence x-ray). In the following weekend, Roentgen ate and slept in his lab (perhaps also to compete with Philipp von Lenard and others who had the same equipment) to repeat the experiments many times, replacing the cardboard with different materials. He found different materials had different abilities to attenuate x-ray. The attenuation increased with material thickness, and lead had the strongest attenuation. In the two weeks following his discovery, he made the first x-ray picture from the hand of his wife (Fig.4.1c), Anna Bertha, which clearly showed her underlying bone structure and her ring. This is the first ever image revealing internal structures of the human body without cutting it open, revolutionizing medicine.

Though x-ray technology has been advanced and standardized to a point where it is used consistently to diagnose and treat patients in modern medicine, it still relies on the same basic principles displayed by Willhelm Rontgen in 1895. X-rays are produced using an X-ray generator, travel through the body part of interest while being attenuated by tissue, and then are detected traditionally by photographic film, and in current digital radiography, by storage-phosphor image plate type digital detector. An X-ray tube consists of a vacuum tube with a cathode and an anode. Modern x-ray tubes use the vacuum and tungsten anode to improve efficiency in generating x-rays. The interaction between x-rays and tissue consists of scattering and absorption and can be characterized by attenuation. Tissue attenuation of x-ray intensity is proportional to tissue density and atomic composition. Typically, x-rays are displayed with higher image intensity for tissue with more attenuation (such as bone and calcified lesions) and lower intensity for tissue with less attenuation (such as soft tissue, air in the lung, and fracture in a bone).

Use of x-ray imaging. Projection x-ray radiography is widely used in the clinic, particularly to visualize dense tissue, such as bone tissue or tumors, or contrasts in dense tissue, such as fractures in bone. For example, an x-ray machine may be used to examine a patient's scoliosis (abnormal curvature of the spine) or to check a patient for breast cancer (mammography). X-ray machines are also used to guide various interventional procedures, which is referred as fluoroscopy (Fig.4.2). An example is fluoroscopy guided coronary angioplasty in the cardiac catheterization suite: a cardiologist inserts a catheter into a femoral artery, moves it to the aorta, then a coronary ostium at the aortic root and then the targeted coronary artery in the heart to deploy a balloon to open the blockage in the artery.

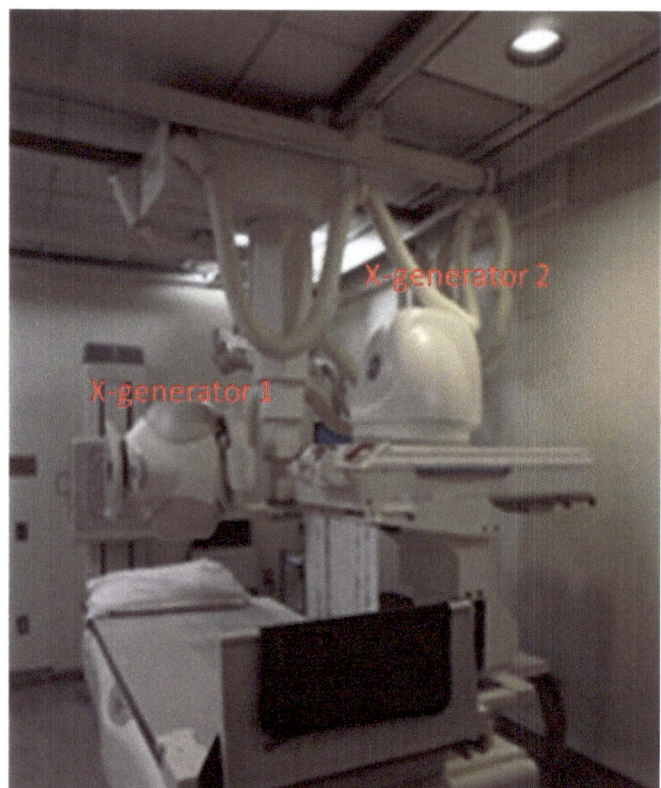

Fig.4.2. A fluoroscopy system using two x-ray generators for horizontal projection (generator 1) and vertical projection (generator 2).

There is some health risk associated with x-ray radiation, which may alter DNA and cause cancer. Low levels of ionizing radiation and infrequent x-ray exposure likely have minimal risk of developing cancer. The amount of x-ray exposure (radiation dose) is monitored by hospital staff working with x-ray equipment and on patients to ensure the risk is very low. However, projection radiography only provides 2D information and lacks depth resolution. This problem is addressed in the development of computed tomography.

4.2   RESOLVING DEPTH – COMPUTED TOMOGRAPHY (CT), AND RELATED POSITRON EMISSION TOMOGRAPHY (PET) AND SINGLE PHOTON EMISSION COMPUTED TOMOGRAPHY (SPECT)

Invention of CT. To generate depth resolution or to create a cross sectional image requires 1) the physics insight that the attenuation detected along a ray is approximately a linear sum of attenuations of all body elements on the ray path and 2) the technical availability to compute the attenuation at each pixel (voxel to be precise, as a ray has thickness). The physics insight may be well known to physicists, and mathematical theories to reconstruct distribution from integral attenuation measurements have been developed in various direct and indirect ways. The basic idea of CT is illustrated in Fig.4.3: measurements from multiple angles are linearly related to attenuations at pixels in the cross section image, and solving this linear system equation allows CT reconstruction. Unfortunately, there was very little impact from people who attacked this problem before enough about computing was known and before computing power was available. Fortunately, after the Second World War, computing power had become available and it was time for the realization of CT. Allan M. Cormack and Godfrey N. Hounsfield, who both knew computing and physics, came across the problem of determining the cross section image of tissue attenuation coefficients at the right time, producing (particularly by Hounsfield) the generally usable CT.

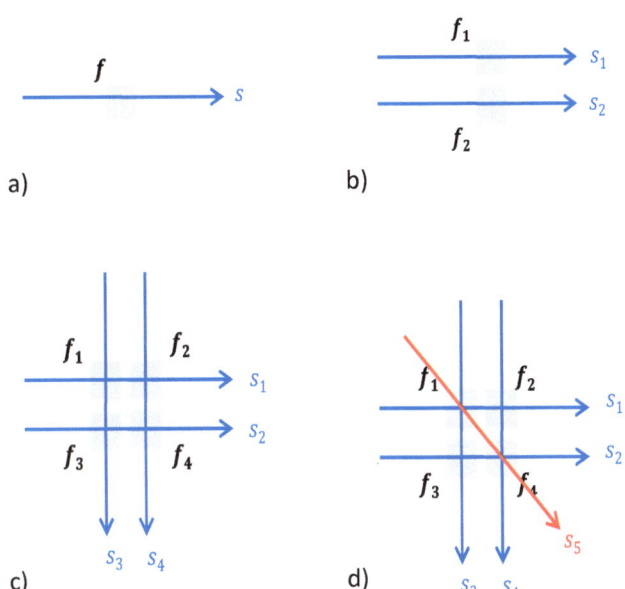

Fig.4.3. The fundamental idea to resolve depth in x-ray. A cross section of an object's x-ray attenuation map is represented by a) 1x1, b)1x2, c)2x2 and d) 2x2 pixels. The attenuation value at each pixel f_j is an unknown. The detector signal (s_i) for each x-ray is a sum of pixel values along the ray $s\_i=\sum\_j [P\_{ij} f\_j]$. The matrix coefficient P_{ij} is determined by the ray path through the object. Therefore, according to linear algebra, to determine an image with NxN pixels, we need NxN measurements – and more (red projection in d), as some of the measurements are not linear independent.

Use of CT. The cross sectional image generated from CT vastly improves the visualization details of internal structures that are buried in projection radiography. The projections at many angles are implemented by rotating the x-ray generator and detectors, and slipper ring technology has been critical for transmission of data and power. A modern CT system (Fig.4.4) typically uses multiple (n=64-256) rows of detectors to image a 3D volume rapidly. CT has a wide range of applications, including identifying intracerebral hemorrhage, lung cancer, and coronary angiography.

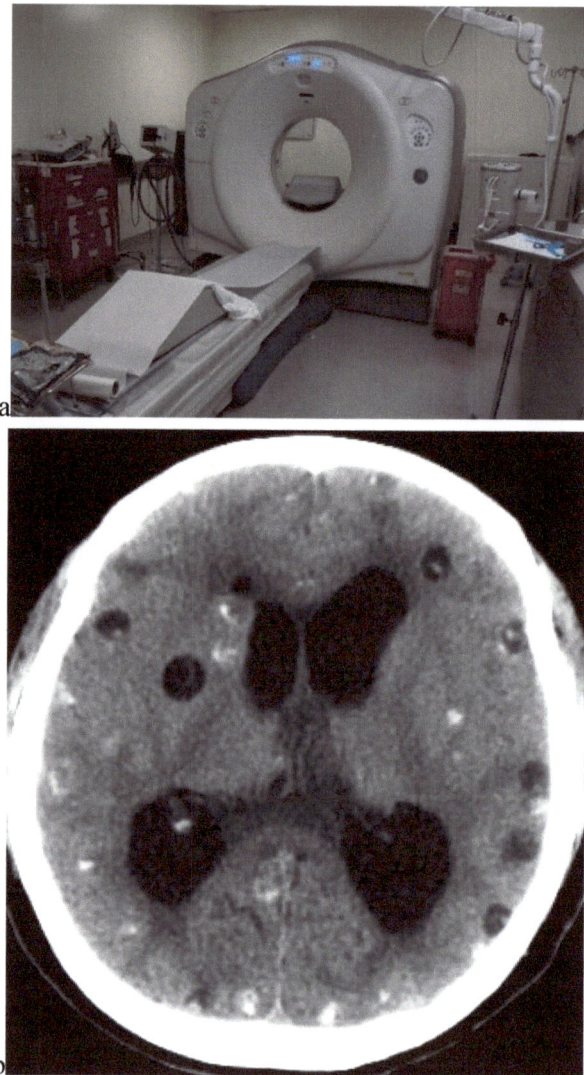

Fig.4.4. a) A CT system; and b) an axial cross section image revealing calcified (bright) and active (dark) lesions in a patient with neurocysticercosis.

Nuclear imaging – PET and SPECT. PET and SPECT are similar to CT but the radiation in PET and SPECT comes from the radioisotope in radioligands or tracers injected into the body. The radioligands participate in biochemistries of the body, typically metabolic activities, revealing tissue functional information and abnormal functions caused by diseases such as tumor and inflammation. PET uses a positron-emitting tracer; the emitted positron annihilates with a nearby electron to produce a pair of gamma photons traveling in opposite directions for detection. There are many PET radioligands being developed by radiochemists to probe various tissue functions. A commonly used PET tracer is fluorodeoxyglucose (FDG), an analogue of glucose that detects metabolic uptake of glucose in tissue. SPECT uses a tracer that emits gamma rays. There are also many SPECT tracers. An example is technetium-99m-tetrofosmin or -sestamibi used in imaging blood flow in myocardium.

The radiation dose issue mentioned in x-ray projection radiography becomes more concerning in CT, which requires many projections. Obviously injecting radioisotopes into the body during PET and SPECT is a concern. This radiation issue (precisely, ionizing radiation) is avoided in two other imaging modalities: magnetic resonance imaging and ultrasound.

4.3   MAGNETIC RESONANCE IMAGING (MRI)

Magnetic resonance physics. MRI is based on the interaction of a magnetic field with body tissue. More than 65% of the human body is composed of water, and each water molecule has two protons. Like a spinning top precesses in the gravity field of earth, a proton experiences a torque in a magnetic field and starts precession around the magnetic field at a frequency proportional to the magnetic field. This is called Larmor precession, with a frequency 128MHz (in radiofrequency range) in a 3T MRI scanner. Larmor precession generates a radiofrequency field that can be detected by a wire loop outside the body, while the proton loses energy. The resting state for the proton in the static 3T field (main magnetic field B0) is to align with the B0 field, experiencing zero torque. A radiofrequency field perpendicular to the B0 field can excite the proton and start precession. This is the magnetic resonance (MR) phenomenon (Fig.4.5a).

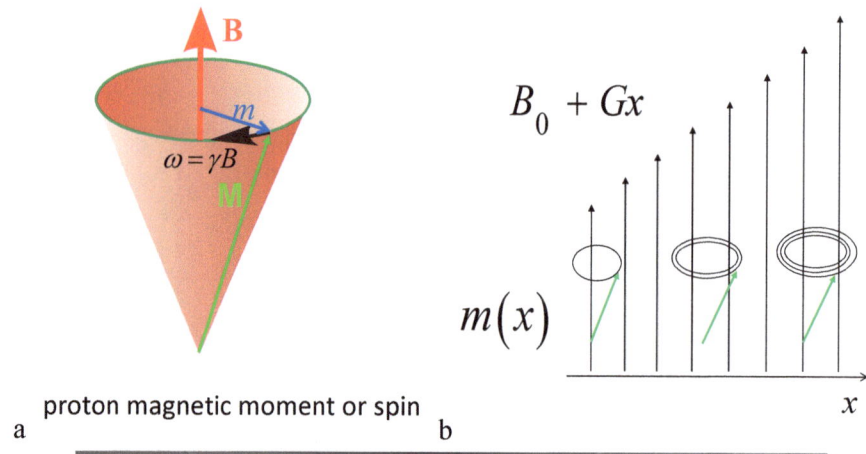

proton magnetic moment or spin

a   b

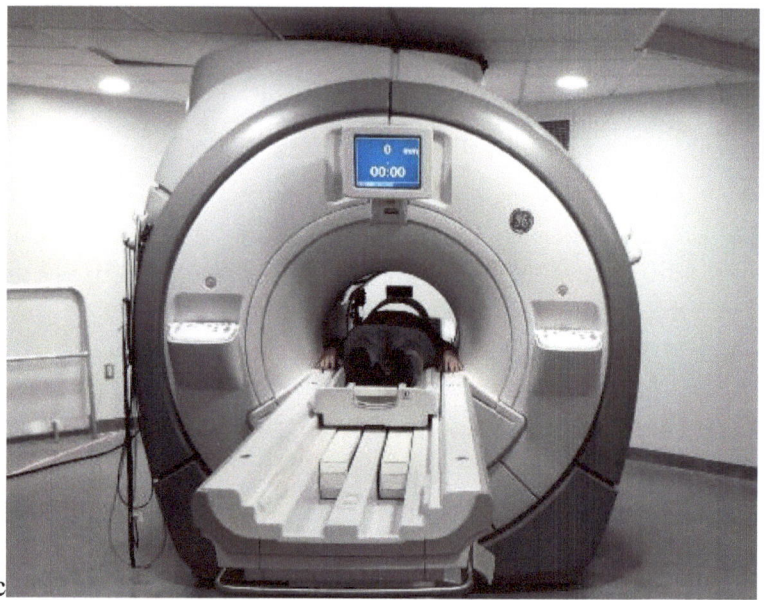

c

Fig.4.5. a) Larmor precession of a proton spin $\mathcal{M}$ in a magnetic field B at a frequency $\omega = \gamma B$. The proportionality constant γ is the gyromagnetic ratio specific to the nucleus (proton here) being investigated. During the Larmor precession, only the spin transverse component m is rotating, which can be characterized by a phase factor $e^{-i\gamma B t}$. b) A gradient field is added to the main magnetic field B0, which makes the Larmor frequency vary linearly in space. Then at a given detection time, the phase factor varies linearly in space ($e^{-i\gamma G x t}$), and the total detected signal $s(t)$ is a sum of all spin contributions weighted by the spatially varying phase factor $s(t) = \sum_x m(x)\, e^{-i(\gamma G t)x}$). This is Fourier transform, or the system matrix is the Fourier encoding matrix. Image can be reconstructed using inverse Fourier transform. c) A 3T MRI system. The "donut" encases the solenoid superconductor coil for B0 field, a gradient coil, and a radiofrequency coil.

Invention of MRI. Magnetic resonance imaging (MRI) was invented right after the invention of CT and uses an approach similar to CT. The MR physics had become well known to physicists and chemists. The computer power had become available for image reconstruction. The time was ready for the birth of MRI, to which many people had contributed. Paul Lauterbur and Peter Mansfield are recognized for the current k-space sampling form of MRI. The linear system matrix connecting the cross section pixel elements and detected signal in CT can be similarly realized in MR by adding a spatial linearly varying magnetic field. This is the gradient field, the core for the invention of MRI, which makes the imaging system matrix a Fourier encoding matrix (Fig.4.5b). MRI can be reconstructed using inverse Fourier transform, which can be executed rapidly using the Fast Fourier Transform (FFT) algorithm (Fig.4.6a). In fact, CT reconstruction is also based on FFT in a modified form. Rapid image reconstruction using an FFT-like algorithm was very important in clinical practice in the early days of CT and MRI when computing power was limited.

Use of MRI. Because proton spin precession is very sensitive to the microenvironment of water, MRI is the method of choice for studying soft tissues, including tissues in the brain, heart, liver, knee, shoulder, etc. Major tissue information in MRI includes the following (Principles of magnetic resonance imaging: physics concept, pulse sequence and biomedical applications. Yi Wang, www.createspace.com):

1) proton thermal microenvironment, which determines water spin T1/T2 relaxation, which largely reflects the cellular contents (macromolecules, membranes, etc.). Approximately, the relaxation rate increases or relaxation times decrease with concentration of cellular contents (macromolecules, membranes, etc.). For example, white matter with highly concentrated myelin (lipid bilayers) has shorter T1 and T2 (darker on T2 weighted ($e^{-TE/T2}$) images and brighter on T1 weighted ($1 - e^{-TR/T1}$) images), compared to gray matter in the brain (Figs.4.6b&c). Here TE is the so-called echo time, and TR the repetition time.
2) transport processes including blood flow, perfusion and diffusion, which affect water spin magnitude and phase.
3) molecular electron cloud's polarization by B0, generating susceptibility field outside the molecule and chemical shift inside the molecule.

Additionally, contrast agents are used to shorten relaxation time and increase magnetic susceptibility.

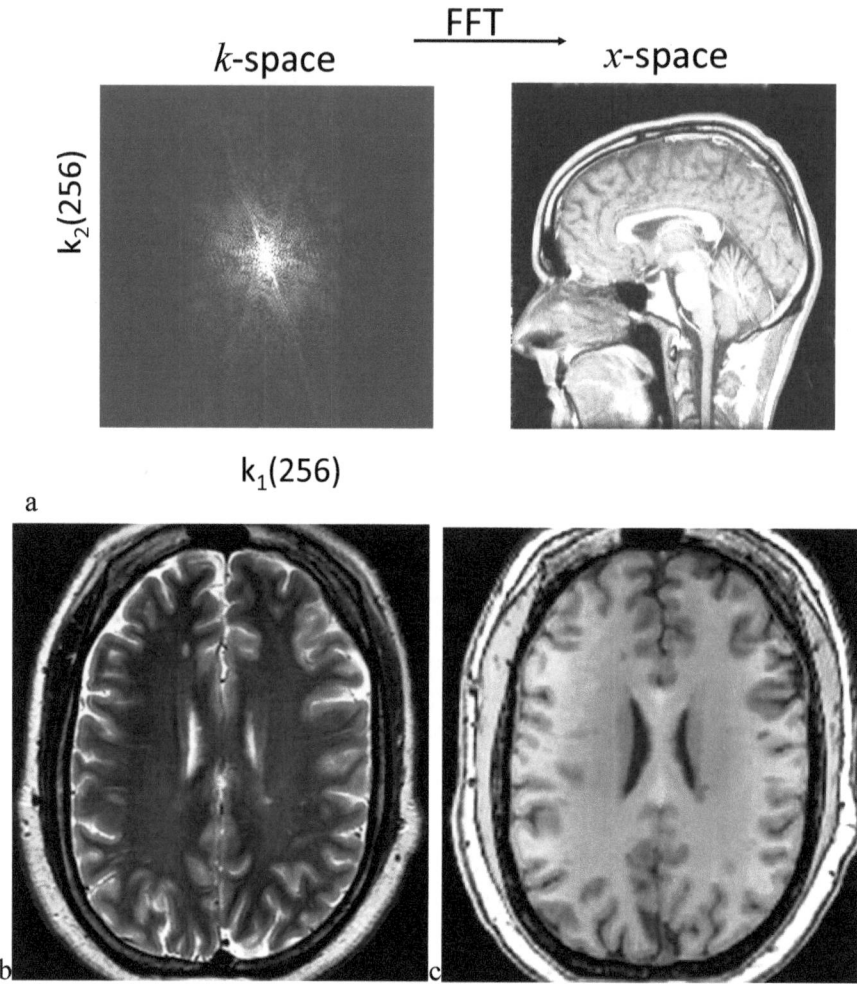

Fig.4.6. a) In MRI, data is acquired in k-space (left). FFT algorithm can rapidly reconstruct image in x-space, showing a sagittal cross section of the brain. Commonly used spine echo images b) with T2 weighting showing bright cerebrospinal fluid (CSF) and gray matter (GM) and dark white matter (WM), and c) with T1 weighting showing dark CSF & GM and bright WM.

Accordingly, there are the following commonly used MRI scans (so called sequences):

1)   T1 and T2 weighted imaging, using the spin echo sequence, are included in almost all MRI protocols in clinical practice. (Spin echo uses 180^0 RF pulse to compensate susceptibility effects and to reveal on relaxation effects, compared to gradient echo.) T2 weighted imaging is used to assess cellular contents in a voxel. For example, loss of myelin content appears as less T2 relaxation decay

or hyperintensity on T2 weighted images (Fig.4.7a). T1 weighted imaging is typically used in conjunction with gadolinium injection and compared with pre-injection to the integrity of the blood brain barrier.

2)   Diffusion weighted imaging sensitized by strong gradients is used to assess tissue damage in ischemic stroke and in tumor; for example, diffusion is reduced in acute ischemia (Fig.4.7b). Diffusion in the brain white matter depends on orientation. Acquisitions using gradients in various directions can be used to form diffusion tension imaging, which are used to study white matter fibers.

3)   Perfusion (blood flow in capillaries) weighted imaging by labeling upstream flowing spins using RF pulses or a contrast agent is used to assess regional tissue blood flow, which is very important for evaluating ischemia and other diseases (Fig.4.7.c).

4)   Magnetic resonance angiography images blood flow in large vessels, which is used to assess vascular diseases (Fig.4.7.d). MRI signal is sensitive to blood flow effects, including time-of-flow effect on signal magnitude, phase contrast effect, and blood contrast enhancement during contrast bolus passage. Contrast agents are sometimes used to enhance relaxation rates of water protons in blood.

5)   T2* weighted imaging using the gradient echo sequence is used to detect magnetic susceptibility abnormalities in tissue caused by blood degradation products, iron deposition, calcification and contrast agents (Fig.4.8). The gradient echo signal magnitude has T2* weighting ($e^{-TE/T2^*}$): 1/T2*=R2* reflects the variance of magnetic field in a voxel multiplied by TE, so T2* weighted hypointensity increases with TE, voxel size and field strength. The gradient echo signal phase reflects the magnetic field multiplied by TE and the gyromagnetic constant: as field is a convolution of tissue magnetic susceptibility with the unit dipole field, deconvolution of the phase can reveal tissue magnetic property.

MRI does not use radiation and is generally considered safe. It is important to avoid bringing ferromagnetic objects close to the magnet, as the main magnetic field can put a very strong force on the ferromagnetic object. Accordingly, contraindications for MRI include various medical implants that may have ferromagnetic components. Currently, most medical implants have been made MRI compatible, which needs to be checked and confirmed on the safety handbook at the MRI scanning console.

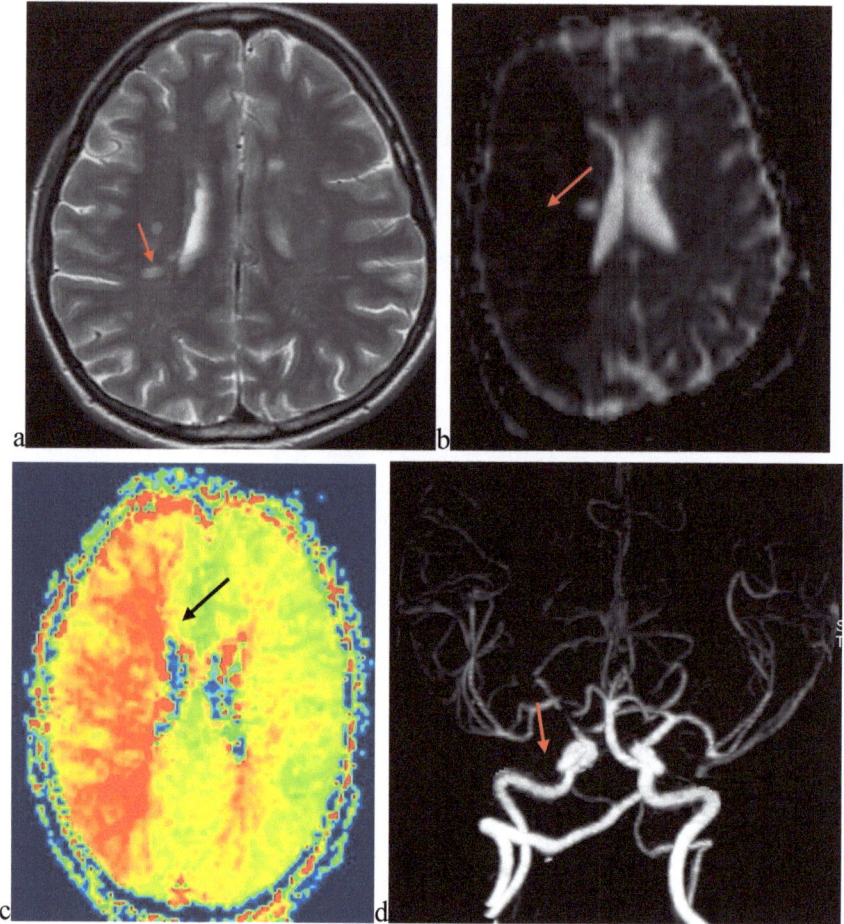

Fig.4.7. Examples of pathologies revealed on MRI (red arrows). a) T2 weighted image of an axial section of the brain showing a hyperintense lesion of multiple sclerosis caused by demyelination (loss of cellular content). b) Diffusion (apparent diffusion coefficient) image showing reduced diffusion in the right side of the brain. c) Perfusion (mean transit time) image showing reduced regional blood flow in the right side of the brain. d) Magnetic resonance angiography (time of flight) demonstrating occlusion of the right mid cerebral arteries of the patient in c.

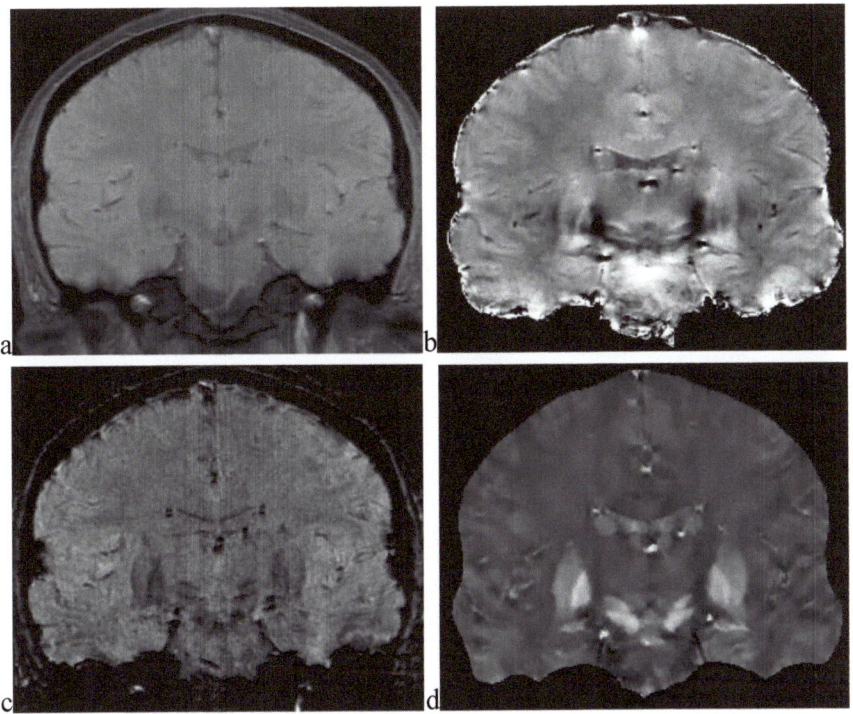

Fig.4.8. Gradient echo imaging sensitizing tissue magnetic susceptibility. a) magnitude image with T2* weighting, b) phase image after unwrapping and background removal, c) susceptibility weighted imaging using additional attenuation based on the phase, and d) quantitative susceptibility mapping (QSM) by deconvolving the phase. Iron depositions in the globus pallidus, subthalamic nucleus and substantia nigra are best depicted on QSM (bright regions).

4.4   ULTRASOUND IMAGING

Basic idea of ultrasound. Sound wave penetration through the body is well known in human history. In fact, the stethoscope (invented in 1816 by Rene Laennec) is a common tool carried around physician's neck to aid the hearing of sound from the patient's heart, lung and other internal organs. Ultrasound is a sound wave with frequency above the human audible range (>20kHz). By the end of the 19th century, it was known that bats use ultrasound to locate/see things, and piezoelectric effects were used to make transducers for generating and detecting ultrasound. Paul Langevin attempted in 1917 to detect a submarine using ultrasound. The idea of ultrasound imaging or echolocation is based on the time of flight in sound wave propagation and reflection (Fig.4.9). Tissue boundaries generate strong sound wave reflection. Scanning using an array of transducers over a range of locations allows formation of an image (vertical positions in Fig.4.9 to form a 2D image, and adding an additional scanning direction for 3D image). A moving object also changes the frequency of the reflected sound wave, which is called the Doppler effect (as in the pitch difference between the approaching and passing siren of an emergency vehicle). Blood flow can be measured from the frequency difference between transmission and echo and is typically displayed in color (Fig.4.10b).

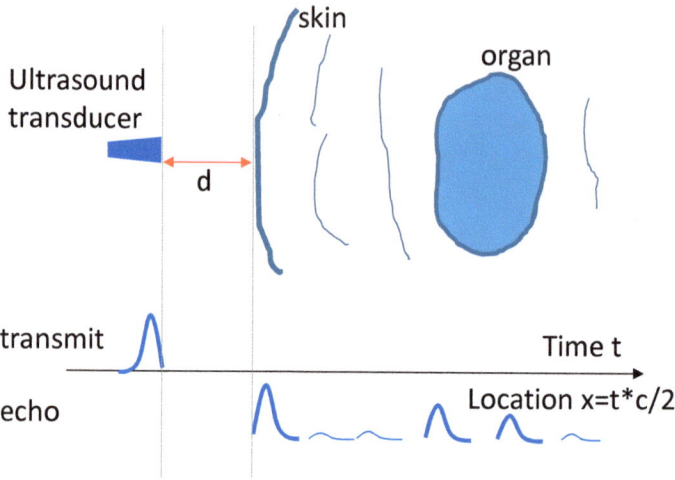

Fig.4.9. Echolocation principle. The location of the reflecting tissue layer is the speed of sound times half the echo time (duration between transmission and echo detection).

Use of ultrasound. Though the image quality of ultrasound is poorer compared to MRI, ultrasound generation and detection is cheaper, faster and more portable than that of MRI. Ultrasound is an important imaging method that does not use radiation, particularly for the dynamic imaging of moving objects. Common uses of ultrasound in hospitals include imaging fetuses in prenatal care, the heart pumping function (Fig.4.10b), bladder function, etc.

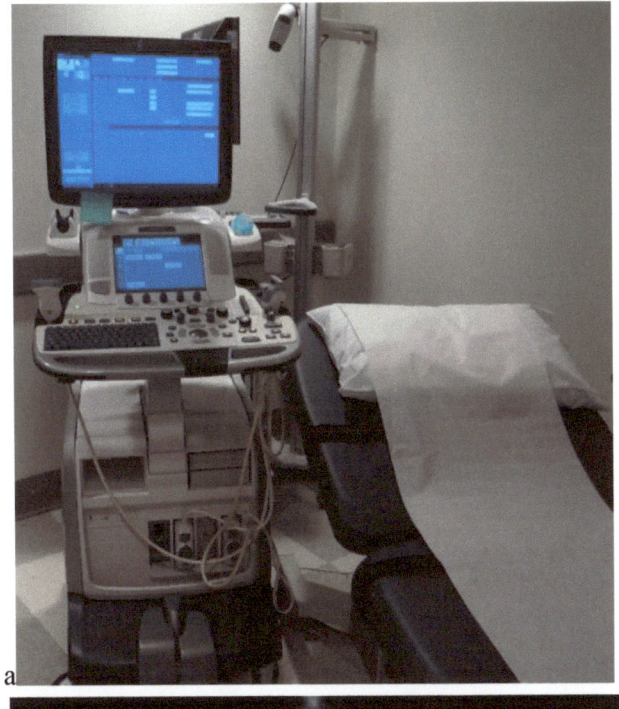

a

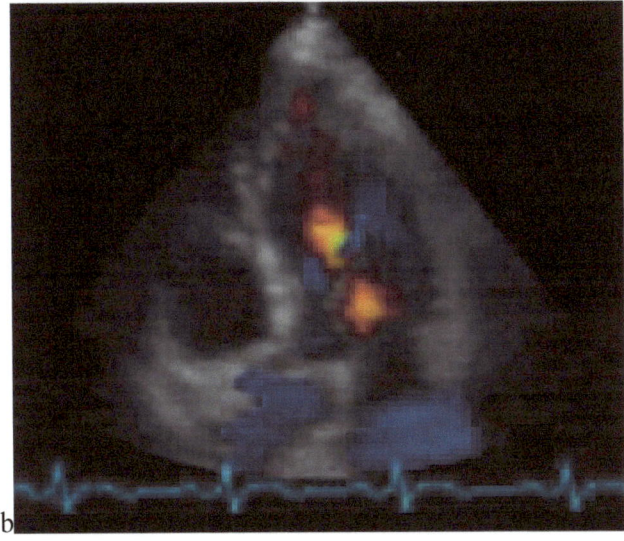

b

Fig.4.10. Ultrasound imaging. a) a typical ultrasound unit. b) An ultrasound image with anatomy of the cardiac chambers and blood flow (in color by the Doppler effect) superimposed.

CHAPTER 5

DIAGNOSIS FROM MEDICAL IMAGES

Zhe Liu and Martin R Prince MD PhD

Once generated by one of the several imaging machines, medical images must be read and interpreted by trained professionals. The correct interpretation of medical images is vital to the execution of effective diagnostic and therapeutic decisions. Reading and interpreting medical images well is a skill that takes many years of training. However, one does not need to be a radiologist to understand the three basic steps of reading medical images: determine the imaging method, understand the scanned anatomy, and locate the abnormal anatomy.

5.1   DETERMINE THE IMAGING METHOD

Various imaging modalities may be used to scan a patient, including x-ray, CT, MRI and ultrasound (US). The first task a radiologist or other health care professional must do when reading an image is to determine the specific method that was used to acquire the image. Though an experienced radiologist can identify the method used to obtain an image without hesitation, this is not a natural skill, but rather one that must be learned and honed through training. Various visual aspects of the imaging methods set them apart from one another. While it is fairly easy to differentiate x-ray, CT and US, the various scanning methods within a modality require expertise to tell apart, particularly so for MRI, which has multiple commonly used contrasts. X-ray radiograph typically displays bone and joint structure as hyper-intense relative to soft tissues. CT scan of the head can visualize calcification and hemorrhage. CT scan of the lung is discernable for the hypointensity of air cavities and hyperintensity of string-like lung vessels and nodular cancerous lesions. MRI has very rich tissue contrasts, as exemplified in the brain case: T1-weighted images show gray matter dark and white matter bright; T2-weighted images show gray matter bright and white matter dark; T2* weighted images show hemorrhage dark; diffusion weighted images show dying cells in acute ischemia as bright. Ultrasound scans are shown in sequential timeframes, with relatively low spatial resolution but superior temporal resolution.

After determining the imaging method, the radiologist must determine what information is expected to be extracted from the image. It is common that X-ray provides skeletal information about bones and joints, and is widely used in examination of chest, hand and limb. CT scans of the lungs reveal information about both acute and chronic changes in the interior of lungs and are always applied to locate lung nodules. MRI, with its ability of various contrast schemes for soft tissues, is widely used for detection and characterization of pathologic lesions in the brain, heart, liver, pancreas and kidneys. Understanding the common principles of basic imaging techniques not only enables us to understand and identify the image method used, but also leads us to deduce the relevant information held in the image.

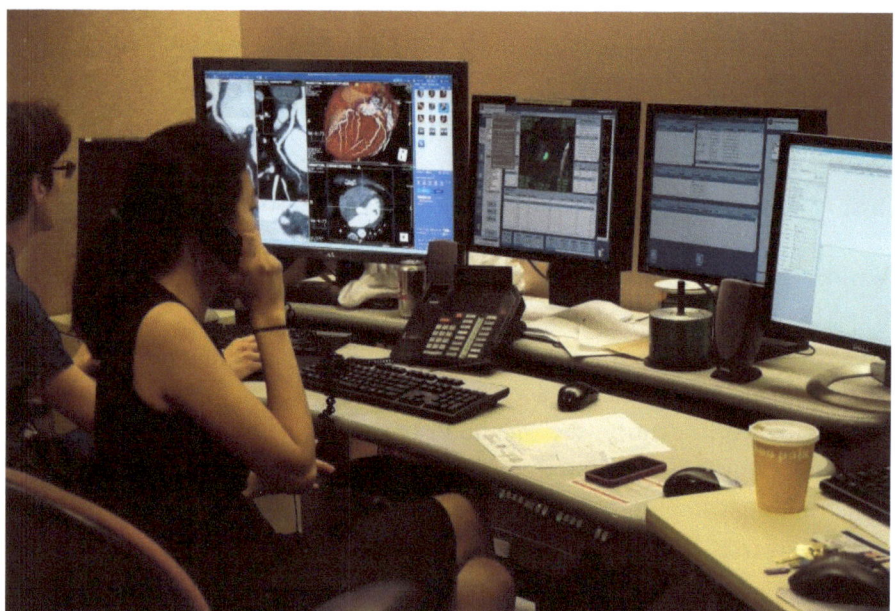

Fig.5.1. Radiologists reviewing images from PACS (picture archive and computing system) on workstations in a radiology reading room.

5.2   UNDERSTAND THE SCANNED ANATOMY

It is essential to understand the anatomical region that is being scanned, i.e., whether it is the head, chest (lung, cardiac), abdominal (liver, spleen, kidney), pelvis (uterus), or a general torso or limb scan. Although with some imaging modalities determining the anatomical context is easy to do, discerning each organ or tissue within the context of the image may be difficult for an inexperienced viewer. One example that illustrates this is an abdominal MRI scan. For this type of scan (Figure 2), it is impossible to make any diagnostic conclusions without a solid understanding of the different regions of the image and to what they correspond.

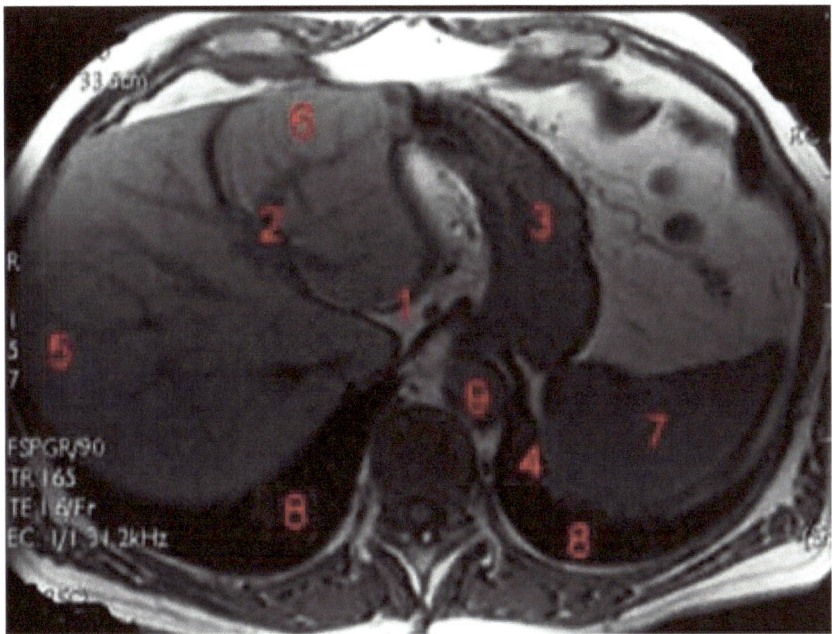

Fig.5.2. Atlas of MR anatomy of abdomen scan: 1: portal hepatis, 2: portal vein, 3: stomach, 4: diaphragm, 5: liver right lobe, 6: liver left lobe, 7: spleen, 8: lung, 9: aorta.

5.3   LOCATE THE ABNORMAL ANATOMY

Locating abnormalities of the anatomy is not only the most important step for determining a diagnosis and potential treatment of a pathology, it is also the most difficult step, requiring years of training before it can be completed proficiently. To diagnose pathology from an image, one must have a thorough understanding of both human anatomy and biochemistry. Additionally, accurate diagnosis requires critical thinking and scientific reasoning, as the radiologist must determine the origin of pathology while provided limited information. The following example is given using an X-ray image of the hand.

In the case of Fig.3, the fifth metacarpal bone is fractured in the transverse direction, while the other metacarpal bones are intact. This fracture is located near the neck of the proximal end of this metacarpal. This type of fracture, which is close to the knuckle, could probably come from the compression of the knuckle against a hard surface, such as a wall or a skull. From the information in the radiograph, it is reasonable to postulate that the patient may have punched his clenched fist against some sort of hard object, which happens frequently among athletes in sports like boxing and martial arts. In fact, this injury is known as "Boxer's fracture".

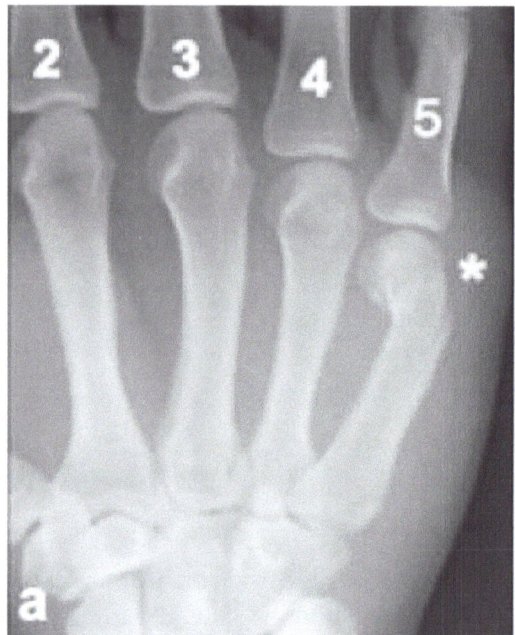

Fig.5.3. X-ray projection radiograph of the Boxer's fracture.

5.4   EXAMPLES ON HOW MEDICAL IMAGING HELPS IN DIAGNOSIS AND TREATMENT PLANNING

Although I had an understanding of how critical medical imaging was to making accurate diagnosis and planning effective treatment, I was still amazed and inspired when observing several real clinical cases, in which radiologists utilized medical images to measure tissue properties, locate pathological sites, guide the therapeutic planning, and examine the quality of treatment.

Case 1: MR Images in Liver Fat Quantification

MR images are normally obtained by exciting tissue in the strong external magnetic field with RF waves, followed by a Fourier spatial encoding scheme and decoding reconstruction. The magnetic moment for tissue is subject to a precession movement in the presence of an external magnetic field (rotation in the transverse plane). Different tissues, such as water and fat, differ in their intrinsic magnetic properties and their magnetic moments (or so-called spins) and therefore rotate with different speed. The signals from different spins are not captured discretely, but rather as a sum. Therefore, at different times the signal may be strong (hyperintense) when the spins of water and fat point to the same direction (called "in-phase" image) or weak (hypointense) when the spins of water and fat have opposite directions (called "out-phase" image, Fig.5.4).

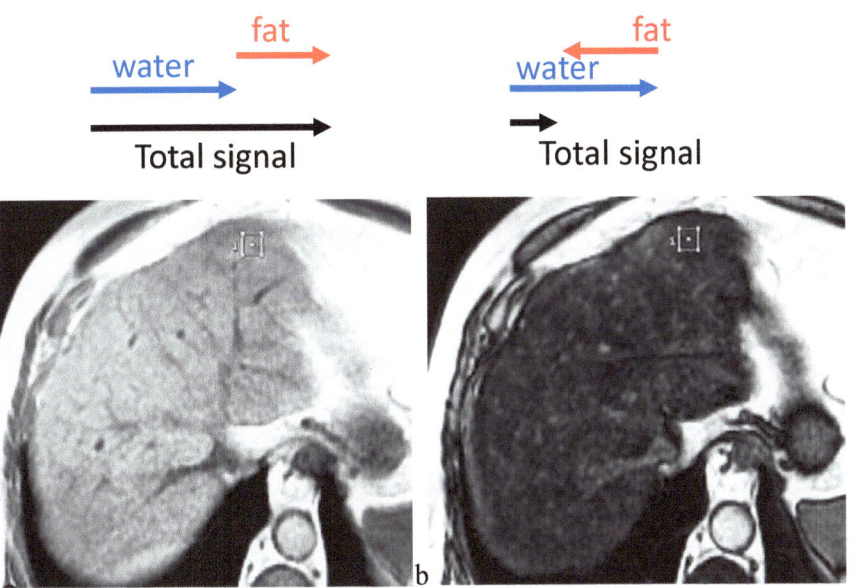

Fig.5.4. Liver imaging using the gradient echo sequence at two different TEs to generate fat-water a) in-phase and b) out-phase images.

With simple algebra, it is possible to obtain the ratio of signal magnitude between water and fat from the pixel intensities in in-phase and out-phase images. Given that the signal for each voxel, which is also proportional to the intensity of the image, is the sum of all spin signals from that voxel, the signal magnitude ratio could reflect the fat percentage in each voxel in the scanned region, e.g. the liver. However, this process is complicated by the fact that spin signals decay in magnitude across different acquisition time points. This problem is usually resolved by comparing the signal reflecting both water and fat to signals from regions with relatively little fat. For example, in an abdominal MR scan, the radiologist typically divides the liver intensity by the spleen intensity in both the in-phase and the out-phase images. This approach is warranted by the fact that the fat content of the spleen is far lower than the fat content of the liver, so the division of the liver intensity by the spleen intensity could be used to compensate for the temporal decay. The following figure shows how radiologists manage to quantify fat content in the liver using in-phase and out-phase abdominal scans.

For each in-phase and out-phase image, radiologists choose regions of interest in the liver and spleen, calculate the intensity average in each region, and divide the mean liver signal intensity by the mean spleen signal intensity. Suppose the ratio is R_{in} for in-phase image, and R_{out} for out-phase image. The liver fat percentage is calculated as $(R_{in}-R_{out})/(2R_{in})*100\%$.

Case 2: Digital Subtraction Angiography in Knee Replacement

Traditional angiography is achieved by injecting an X-ray opaque contrast agent into the patient's blood vessel and then using X-ray imaging. The contrast enhanced X-ray image shows the contrast of the blood vessels against the background, but other structures such as bones and joints are also discernable. In order to get rid of the structures besides the blood vessels, Digital Subtraction Angiography is employed by subtracting the contrast enhanced image by a "mask image", which is taken at the same region before the injection of the contrast agent. The resultant image displays the blood vessels and their surrounding gray background with superior contrast. This technique is often used to examine blood vessels in knee replacement treatment, in which the post-operative growth of blood vessels around the implant site is critical for replacement success (Fig.5.5).

During my hospital experience, I witnessed a knee replacement case in which the patient was given a knee replacement made of metal and plastic that led to his return to the hospital due to severe swelling around the implant. The area around the implant was mostly filled with blood and the preliminary diagnosis was hyper-vascularity. In order to remove the over-growing blood vessels, physicians needed to know the exact location of the vessels. This information was obtained using Digital Subtraction Angiography, in which the doctor injected iodine contrast into the artery at the root of the thigh (where the artery is close to the skin), and took knee X-ray images at the rate of 10 per sec. Because the contrast in the blood vessels is opaque on X-ray, subsequent images are subtracted for better vascular visualization. Using this technique, the doctor could easily discern the location of the over-grown vascularity and effectively treat the pathology.

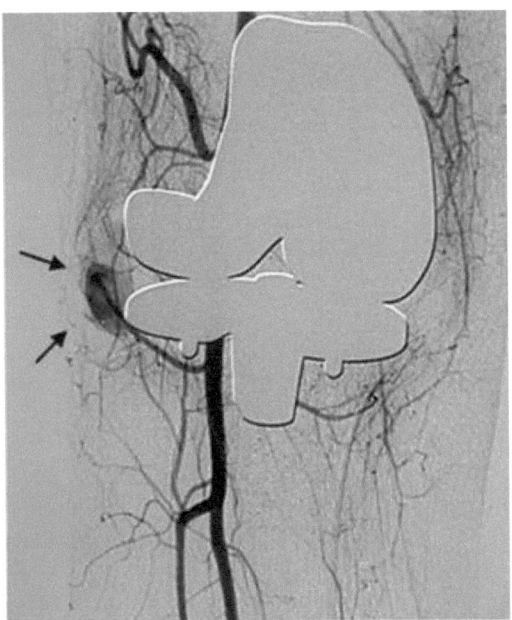

Fig.5.5. Example of digital subtraction angiography at knee implant site. Area for suspected aneurysm of the inferior medial popliteal artery is observed from the image (Swiss Med Wkly. 2010;140:w13094).

CHAPTER 6

BASIC MEDICAL DEVICES – SURGICAL TOOLS

Andrew Luzzi

During the Clinical Summer Immersion program at Cornell University, the Biomedical Engineering students witnessed numerous operations and observed the variety of instruments and devices used in surgical procedures. The completion of one surgery typically involves many steps and different techniques, and, as such, a multitude of surgical equipment exists to aid the surgeon in whatever task is required. A myriad of surgical tools are currently used in modern medicine, but many can be organized based on function. This chapter will examine the basics of surgical equipment.

6.1 TOOLS TO CUT TISSUE AND EXPOSE THE BODY

Many surgical tools are simple instruments that allow the surgeon to mechanically manipulate tissue. The scalpel, a staple of the surgeon's arsenal, comes in various shapes and sizes but always consists of a handle and a blade. It is commonly used for initial incisions, as well as cutting through deeper skin layers, muscle, and fat. Surgical scissors, like scalpels, are also used for cutting through skin, muscle, and fat. They resemble standard scissors, but are often smaller so they may be manipulated in limited space and sharper so they may cut through tissue with less resistance.

In order to grasp and manipulate tissue so that it may be dissected, forceps are used. The term forceps can refer to instruments that look like what are commonly referred to as "tweezers" or may refer to instruments that superficially resemble scissors, but instead of sharp blades forceps have a variety of non-cutting appendages to use for various purposes. Duval's forceps, for example, have wide and dull extensions to minimize trauma when grasping delicate tissue such as stomach or lung.

Clamps are a subset of surgical forceps which have a handle mechanism that allows surgeons to lock the appendages closed. These are frequently used to clamp blood vessels during operations. Retractors, on the other hand, are used by surgeons to separate the edges of an incision. Some retractors are simple and consist of a hooked blade with a handle, others are similar to scissors and possess two dull curved blades that can be spread apart, and others are more complicated still. Regardless of their appearance, retractors are used to spread more superficial tissue apart so that the underlying tissue can be viewed. These tools are the basic surgical instruments used to cut, clamp, separate, and maneuver different tissue throughout an operation.

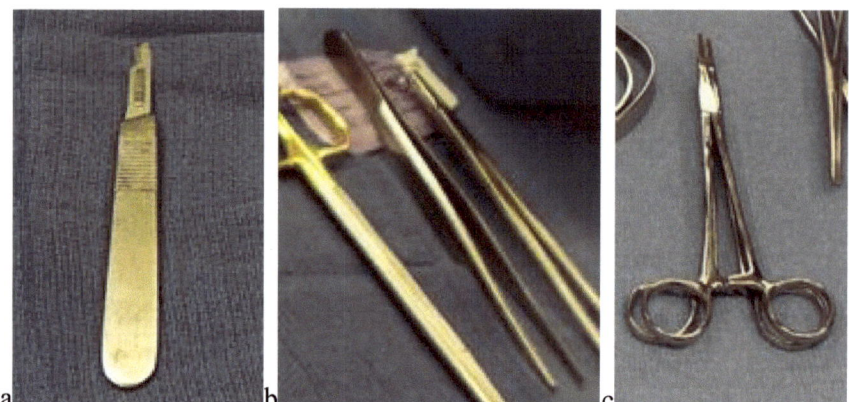

Fig.6.1. a) Scalpel. b) Forceps. c) Surgical Scissors.

6.2   HIGH-TECH TOOLS FOR TISSUE MANIPULATION

In addition to these instruments, there are many more technologically advanced devices being used to manipulate and expose tissue as well. One device, termed a laser scalpel, uses laser light to cut through tissue. The light is typically produced by running an electric current through a specific type of gas and the frequency of the light produced varies depending on the gas used. Different frequencies of light, produced using different gases, have distinct functions in surgery. A CO_2 laser produces infrared light and is used to ablate   soft   tissue   with   high   water   content,   such   as   fat. (**http://www.intechopen.com/books/co2-laser-optimisation-and-application**) An **excimer** laser, which uses a dimeric or heterodimeric molecule that decays and releases electromagnetic radiation, produces light in the ultra violet range and is used for eye surgeries. Using lasers can be advantageous for several reasons. Notably, lasers cauterize blood vessels as they cut and thus minimize the amount of bleeding that occurs during an operation. Additionally, lasers make very precise cuts and therefore minimize unnecessary damage to healthy tissue.

Though not as delicate as lasers, drills also have several surgical applications. Drills are used primarily to penetrate hard, dense tissue such as bone. Many neurosurgical procedures require the use of a drill to penetrate the skull and

66

expose the underlying brain and many orthopedic procedures require drills to facilitate the implantation of screws into bone.

Arthroscopic shavers are another motorized tool that serve multiple functions in surgery. A shaver consists of a long, hollow steel rod with a rotating blade at one end. When the surgeon squeezes the rotating hand piece attached to the arthroscopic shaver, the blade rotates. The rotating blade not only sheers and cuts tissue, but also, due to the suction created by the rotation, sucks detached tissue into the blade and away from the area of operation. The arthroscopic shaver is ideal for shaving loose tissue and clearing debris from surgical sites.

6.3   WOUND CLOSURE

While scalpels, drills, and lasers can expose the body for surgery, in order to close wounds resulting from surgery, trauma, or pathology, other devices must be used. The most basic sealing device is the suture. Surgical sutures, consisting of a needle and a thread and colloquially referred to as stiches, differ from the common stich in several ways. Surgical sutures are made from a variety of natural sources, such as collagen and stainless steel, and synthetic sources, such as Nylon and Polysorb, and have a number of variable characteristics. The ideal suture has flexibility, high tensile strength, and the ability to hold when knotted. Additionally, ideal sutures are resistant to infection and cause minimal tissue reaction. Composed of several filaments, a multifilament suture is more flexible and has higher tensile strength than a monofilament suture. However, monofilament sutures, which retain less water than multifilament sutures, typically elicit a lower tissue reaction.

Additionally, all sutures can be classified as either absorbable or non-absorbable. Absorbable sutures degrade in the body over time and can be beneficial to close internal wounds, eliminating the need to re-open the patient, or close superficial wounds, eliminating the need to take out the sutures. Non-absorbable sutures do not degrade in the body and are typically used to close wounds that have a lengthy healing period. Additionally, modern sutures are hypoallergenic, thus preventing allergic reactions to the suture, and many are also coated with antimicrobial substances to mitigate infection.

Tissue adhesives, made from cyanoacrylates – the same compound from which super glues are derived, can be used to repair small and superficial wounds and lacerations. Modern tissue adhesives are able to be stored and applied in liquid form. Upon contact with the skin (or other water containing substances), the adhesive polymerizes, creating an anti-microbial seal over the wound. Using tissue adhesives to close wounds eliminates the discomfort associated with the input of sutures. The use of tissue adhesives also eliminates the suture removal process and typically saves time.

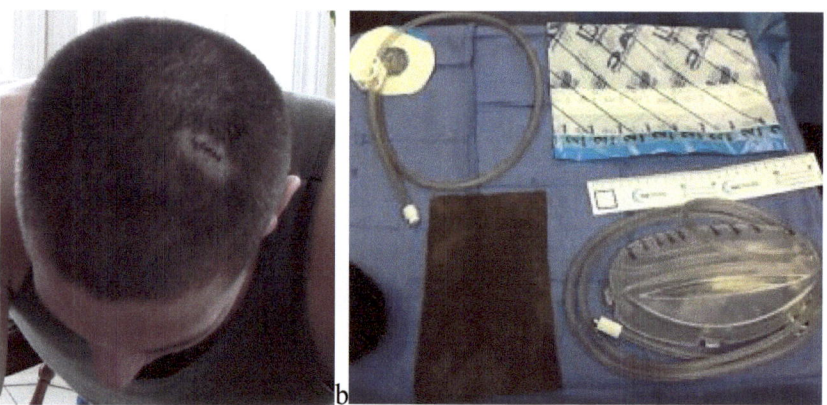

Fig.6.2. a) Sutures used to close head laceration. b) Materials for vacuum assisted wound closure.

Vacuum-Assisted Closure, pioneered by plastic surgeons at Wake Forest, is a recent technological advance in the treatment of wounds. While able to treat acute wounds, this method is more typically used for chronic wounds and burns. In vacuum-assisted closure, also referred to as negative pressure wound therapy, a piece of foam is initially fitted and placed into the wound and an adhesive membrane is then placed on top of the foam. A drainage tube is fitted through an opening in the film in order to collect fluids. Fitted through another hole in the film, a vacuum pump creates a partial vacuum in the wound by applying negative pressure to the location. The adhesive membrane prevents the inflow of air, which would disrupt the vacuum, and the foam helps to expose every part of the wound to a uniform negative pressure. The vacuum is believed to "[assist] with the removal of interstitial fluid, decreasing localized oedema and increasing blood flow." **http://www.worldwidewounds.com/2001/may/Thomas/Vacuum-Assisted-Closure.html**

Replacement skin and skin like substances can also be used to repair skin trauma. Autologous skin grafts, where the skin is grafted from a different place on the same individual, and allogenic skin grafts, where the skin is grafted from another person, typically a cadaver, have been used extensively to treat skin trauma, but have several disadvantages. Autologous skin grafts may be disadvantageous because of the limiting amount of skin able to be grafted from the patient, and allogenic skin grafts may result in rejection by the patient or rejection. To improve treatment of skin trauma, synthetic skin has been developed. The type of synthetic skin can vary, but most is composed of a collagen scaffold that is often seeded with the patient's own cells. Applied so that it covers the wound, artificial skin promotes the growth of new skin cells and protects the patient from dehydration and infection. Many aspects of artificial skin and its application are currently being investigated and tested, and it is possible that spray on skin, skin created from spider silk scaffolds, and skin that uses semiconductors to sense touch will be used in the clinic in the future.

http://news.discovery.com/tech/artificial-skin-spider-silk-110810.htm

While sutures and adhesives close superficial wounds, bone cement is used to close gaps inside the body related to artificial joints. When a prosthesis is surgically inserted and attached to a bone, a free space exists between the bone and prosthesis. This free space is filled with bone cement, which serves the functions of both anchoring the prosthesis to the bone and increasing the absorptive ability of the artificial joint. Bone cement initially consists of two phases, one powder, frequently PMMA based, and one liquid, frequently an MMA monomer, which are mixed together. One of the phases typically contains an initiator, and upon mixing, free radical polymerization occurs and the viscosity of the cement steadily increases. The cement is applied as a viscous, doughy, liquid and eventually hardens into a solid.

http://www.scielo.br/scielo.php?script=sci_arttext&pid=S0104-66322011000200007

6.4   MINIMALLY INVASIVE TRANSLUMINAL DEVICES

A relatively recent advancement in surgery, endoscopic techniques have spawned many minimally invasive surgical procedures along with various new pieces of surgical equipment. Endoscopic surgery refers to surgical procedures in which a scope is inserted through a natural body opening or a small incision. Minimally invasive procedures have several advantages, including in many cases a decreased risk of infection, a faster recovery, and a smaller scar. The staple of endoscopic procedures is the endoscope. The endoscope has a flexible shaft that, on one end, has a camera and a light. This part of the endoscope is inserted into the body and allows the physician to view the desired internal area of the patient. The images of objects are typically relayed to the eyepiece on the handle of the endoscope using fiber optics or are projected onto a screen using a camera. In addition to frequently containing an eyepiece, the handle of the endoscope also has controls that allow the physician to manipulate the part of the scope that is being inserted into the patient. In order to perform additional medical functions, the endoscope has a channel through which other medical instruments can be inserted. It is through the joint functions of visualization and a combination of cutting, shaving, and manipulating tissue that the endoscope enables a physician to repair torn joint tissue, remove impaired gall bladders, perform bypass surgery, and treat various other medical conditions in a minimally invasive fashion.

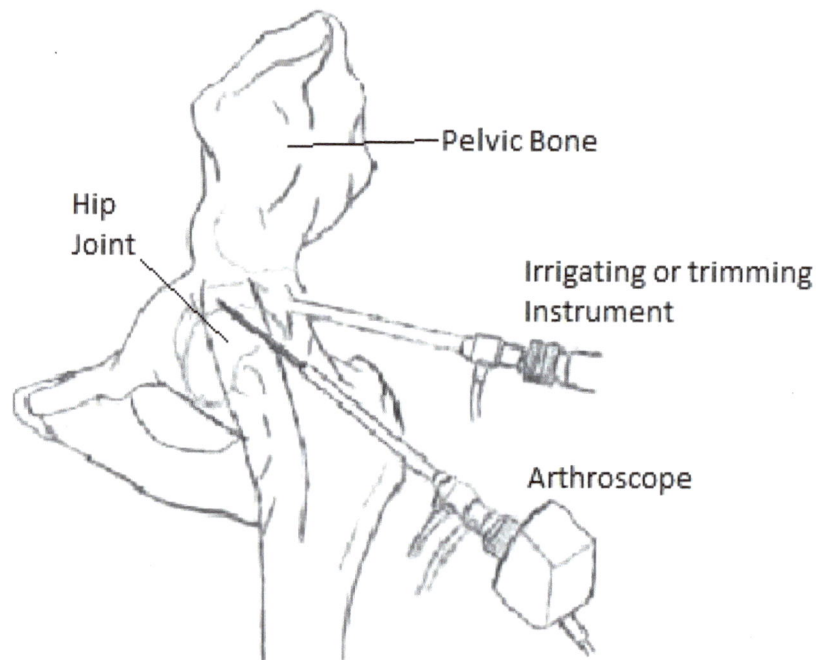

Fig.6.3. Hip Arthroscopy

6.5   ROBOTIC SURGERY

In addition to endoscopic techniques, robotic surgery has recently become more popular and has revolutionized the way various operations are performed. Robotics are used to operate in order to reduce the amount of human error involved in surgery. Through several methods, robotic surgery provides the benefit of clean, quantified surgical movements, the preciseness of which cannot be obtained using exclusively a human hand. The exactness of robotic surgery allows for smaller incisions, more efficient cuts, and the option to perform some surgeries using minimally invasive technique that

70

previously required open technique. These advantages of robotic surgery can lead to less blood loss, less tissue damage, smaller scars, and a shorter recovery time. One method of robotic surgery uses a telemanipulator, which involves a pair of robotic arms performing the surgery and a surgeon controlling the arms by carrying out typical surgical movements. Another method, appropriately deemed computer-controlled surgery, involves a surgeon using a computer to control the actions of the robotic arms. Valve repairs, pancreatectomies, hysterectomies, joint replacements, and many other surgeries in various surgical specialties have been performed with the assistance of robotics. Despite some clear advantages of robotic surgery, it also tends to cost more and the long term health benefits of robotic vs. non robotic surgery are not conclusive. Regardless, robotic surgery remains a viable method of performing many surgeries today and there is no doubt that with increasing technological advancement the scope and effectiveness of robotic surgery will continue to increase in the future.

6.6   IRRIGATION AND DRAINAGE

During many surgical procedures, fluids are introduced and/or removed from operation sites. An irrigator is used to flush a wound or operation site with fluid. The passing of fluid over an operation or wound site clears away debris, which both improves visibility and discards material that could be disruptive to the surgeon or pathogenic in nature. The irrigation fluid may also be used to achieve wound hydration. When irrigating a wound, the irrigation equipment, the method of irrigation, the composition of irrigation solution, and the pressure at which the irrigation solution is kept are all taken into consideration. Bulb syringes and piston syringes are two cost effective pieces of equipment that can facilitate wound irrigation. However, the low pressure provided by these syringes may not be as effective at clearing debris and decreasing bacterial load. More elaborate devices that provide pulsed, high pressure irrigation are frequently high cost and cumbersome. Pressurized canisters are also viable pieces of equipment to facilitate the irrigation of wounds. These canisters are relatively inexpensive and can provide high pressure irrigation, however the canister reliability and the warming of the solution in the canister to room temperature can be problematic.

Irrigation solution, in addition to other fluids such as blood, saliva, and other bodily secretions, must frequently be removed from the patient's body during surgery in order improve visibility and clear debris and pathogens. Many hospitals have central vacuum systems, which involve the creation of a vacuum by a device somewhere in the hospital. Many tubes are connected to this device and are directed to other rooms in the hospital, such as operating rooms. In the operating room, a surgeon is able to connect a variety of instruments to the tubing of the central vacuum system. The specific instrument to be used depends on the specific task that must be accomplished. A surgeon may use a thin, smaller instrument called a Frazier suction tip when dealing with small surgical settings. A larger instrument, called a Yankauer suction tip, may be used for larger surgical settings.

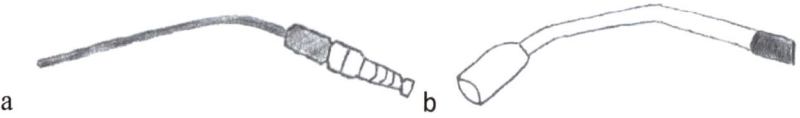

Fig.6.4. a) Frazier Suction Tip. b) Yankauer Suction Tip.

6.7   CONCLUSION

A vast array of surgical equipment exists to assist surgeons in the execution of the many different surgical procedures. This chapter covers some basic categories of surgical equipment, but many medical tools and devices not mentioned in this chapter exist and have important clinical uses. With perpetual technological and medical advancement arises the unremitting demand for improved and novel medical devices, notably surgical equipment. Biomedical engineers, being at the forefront of the development of novel medical technology, must have a solid grasp of the current and potential future environment of surgical equipment in order to be best prepared to make significant technological advancements.

CHAPTER 7

BASIC SURGICAL TREATMENT EXEMPLIFIED BY THYROID SURGERY

Andrew Luzzi and Frank Luzzi MD

This chapter will illustrate how surgery can be used to treat a pathological condition by detailing the surgical management of a thyroid nodule. The chapter will describe the initial diagnosis, the factors contributing to the decision for surgery, the logistics of the operating room, and the surgical procedure itself.

7.1   BASIC THYROID ANATOMY AND FUNCTION

The thyroid is an endocrine gland found in the neck. It produces the hormones triiodothyronine and thyroxine, which affect a vast array of metabolic, developmental, and homeostatic processes of the body.

The following is a basic outline of thyroid structure and other related anatomy. The thyroid consists of two lobes with vertically oriented axes that are connected by an isthmus. The top part of a lobe is called the superior pole and the bottom part of a lobe is called the inferior pole. The thyroid is located in the anterior (front) lower neck and is attached to the underlying trachea by two ligaments called Berry's Ligaments. Four small endocrine glands, called parathyroid glands, modulate calcium levels in the body and are physically associated with the thyroid gland but not affiliated metabolically. The superior parathyroid glands are found along the posterior superior surface, and the inferior thyroid glands are adjacent to the inferior poles of the thyroid. Several important blood vessels and nerves are also in close proximity to the thyroid.

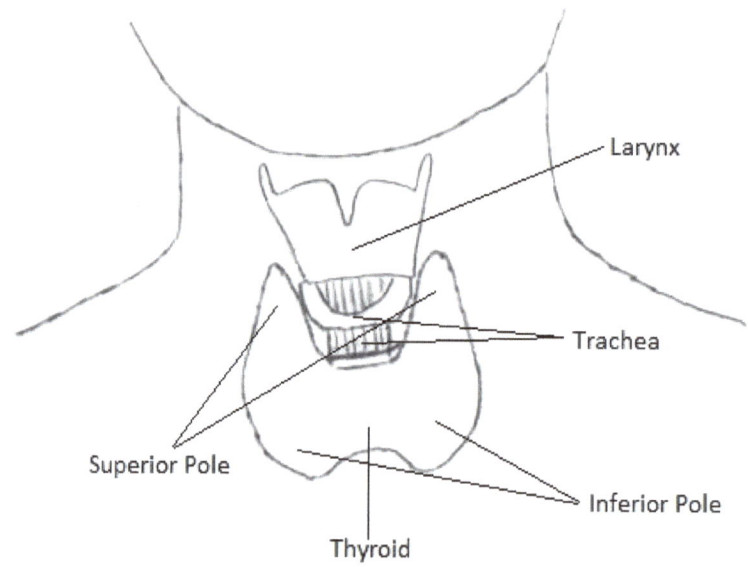

Fig.7.1. Basic Thyroid Anatomy.

7.2   DIAGNOSIS OF A THYROID NODULE

A thyroid nodule may initially be suspected when a patient feels a lump in their lower neck, a physician feels the lump during a routine physical exam, or a physician finds the nodule on a radiologic exam for an unrelated problem. In any case, the physician will palpate the thyroid with the patient swallowing and not swallowing. Swallowing shifts the gland superiorly, at times allowing a better evaluation of the nodule. If the physician determines that there is a problem, an ultrasound of the gland will be performed to confirm the nodule's presence. If the nodule appears on this exam to have concerning features, such as calcifications, a certain minimal size, usually 5mm, or a complex nature (part solid and part cystic), a fine needle aspiration biopsy will be ordered. This biopsy of the nodule will be sent for cytologic evaluation. The cytology results will dictate the treatment taken. If the nodule is felt to be benign, the thyroid may continue to be monitored or no further evaluation may be required. If the cytology shows concerning features, such as atypia of the genetic material, monitoring or surgical intervention will be decided upon. If there is a strong suspicion for cancer, surgery will be recommended.

This chapter will assume that the patient has a 1.5cm nodule in the right thyroid lobe having concerning features but not outright malignant changes on cytology. The physician will then discuss the option of a right hemi thyroidectomy with the patient and its associated risks and benefits. The physician will explain to the patient that the right side of the thyroid, once removed, will be sent to the pathology department while the patient is still on the operating room table to determine if the nodule is cancerous. The pathologist will determine whether or not the nodule is a cancer and will relay this information back to the operating room and surgeon. If the nodule is cancerous, the surgeon may then remove the remaining thyroid gland.

7.3   PRE-SURGICAL TREATMENT AND PLANNING

Before the patient undergoes surgery, he must have several tests. The physician will ensure that the vocal cords are performing normally by mirror or fiber optic exam. Vocal cord function can be compromised by the cancer itself or by trauma during the surgery. Additionally, prior to the surgery, laboratory tests will determine the baseline level of thyroid and parathyroid function. Specifically, thyroid stimulating hormone level, which correlates to thyroid function, and ionized calcium level, which correlates to parathyroid function, will be measured. Thyroid function is often reduced proportionately to the amount of thyroid surgically removed. Parathyroid function may be impaired, as the glands are so small and intimately associated with the thyroid that they may be directly damaged, their vasculature may be compromised, or at times they may be removed inadvertently during surgery.

Also prior to the surgery, the physician will outline the risks of the operation to the patient. These include risks of bleeding, infection, and scar formation, risk of damage to the nerves that supply the voicebox, and risk of damage to the parathyroid glands.

7.4   SURGICAL CARE

The patient is brought into the operating room and general anesthesia induced. The patient is intubated with an endotracheal tube that has electrodes that connect to a nerve integrity monitor and are positioned at the level of the vocal cords. If the nerve that innervates the muscles to the vocal cords, the recurrent laryngeal nerve, is manipulated during surgery, the vocal cord will move and the electrodes will send a signal to the nerve integrity monitor which will alert the surgeon with an audible beep. The importance of this device will be highlighted later in the chapter.

The surgeon scrubs his hands with antibacterial soap outside of the operating room. Upon entering the operating room, the surgeon dons a gown, gloves, and a headlight with assistance from the nurses. The patient is positioned in a neck extended position. This means that the chin is up and the head is back. This position is achieved with the help of a roll positioned beneath the shoulders of the patient. This position elongates the neck and makes the thyroid easier to access. After cleaning the neck with alcohol, the surgeon palpates the thyroid notch and approximately two finger breadths superiorly draws a gently curved line with a marker in a natural skin crease extending from one sternocleidomastoid muscle to the other. This demarcation is then injected with 1% lidocaine with a dilution of 1:100,000 epinephrine to provide a local anesthetic and vasoconstrictive effect. The patient is prepped with betadine extending from the chin to the superior aspect of the chest and as far lateral right and left as possible. Then, sterile drapes are placed to isolate the field of interest – the anterior neck.

As the nodule is in the right thyroid lobe, the surgeon approaches the operating table and stands on the patient's right. Across from the surgeon is his assistant. To the surgeon's right stands the scrub nurse, who will hand equipment to the surgeon throughout the case.

7.5   THE OPERATION, PART 1: OBTAINING EXPOSURE TO THE SURGICAL FIELD

The surgeon makes an incision along the line of demarcation, cutting sequentially through skin, subcutaneous tissue, and the platysma muscle (a superficial muscle covering most of the neck) with a sharp, steel knife. The platysma muscle is invested in fascia – a fibrous connective tissue. Beneath this fascia, the surgeon uses electrocautery or sharp scissors to separate this flap of skin, subcutaneous tissue, muscle, and fascia from the underlying structures of the neck, both superiorly and inferiorly. These flaps are then retracted using retaining sutures. The surgeon has now gained exposure to what will be the surgical field.

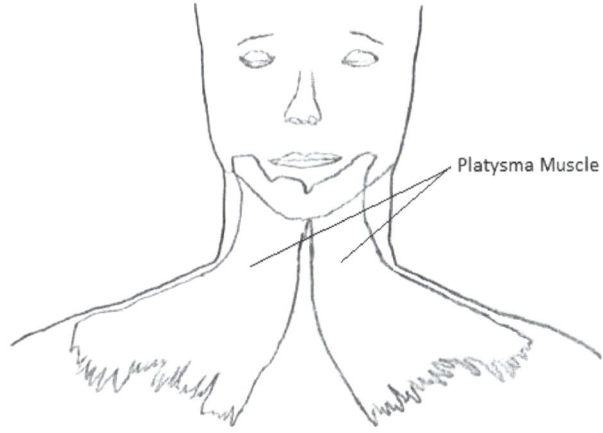

Platysma Muscle

Fig.7.2. The Platysma Muscle.

7.6   THE OPERATION, PART 2: ISOLATING THE RIGHT THYROID LOBE AND LOCATING THE RECURRENT LARYNGEAL NERVE

What the surgeon initially sees are strap muscles – a group of four pairs of muscle in the anterior part of the neck covering the trachea, cricoid cartilage, and larynx. The linea alba refers to a line that separates the left and right strap muscles. The surgeon begins the second part of the operation by grasping the midline of the strap muscles just below the cricoid cartilage in an attempt to locate the linea alba. Then sharply, the linea alba is incised, separating the strap muscles right and left. The surgeon then bluntly retracts the strap muscles and separates them from the underlying thyroid gland. For this particular case, this is primarily done on the right side, leaving the left thyroid lobe only partially visible.

Attention is then directed at the superior thyroid pole. An Army-Navy retractor is placed under the superior flap, and strong retraction is often required to expose the pole. The surgeon will gently dissect overlying tissues away from the superior pole of the thyroid using a clamp with a spreading action or a fine piece of cotton held in a clamp in a pushing fashion. He will then, with the same instruments, isolate the superior thyroid artery and vein. Once done, these vessels are separately clamped, incised, and ligated, often using right angled clamps. The surgeon is careful not to extend his dissection beyond the superior extent of the thyroid, so as not to damage the nearby superior laryngeal nerve, which innervates the cricothyroid muscle that tenses the vocal cords.

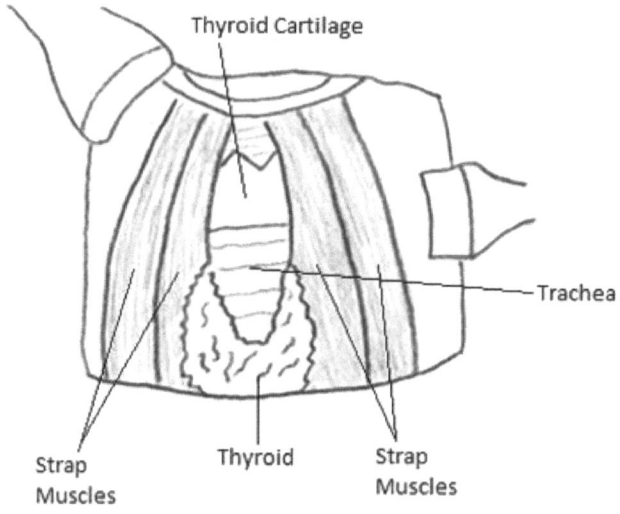

Fig.7.3. Strap Muscles in Relation to Trachea and Thyroid.

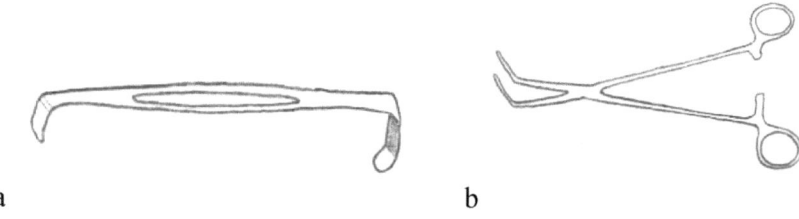

a   b

Fig.7.4. a) Army-Navy Retractor. b) Kelly Clamp.

Next, attention is directed at the lateral aspect of the thyroid lobe, where blunt dissection is utilized to isolate the middle thyroid vein. Once done, this vein is double clamped, incised, and ligated as close to the capsule of the gland as possible. During this dissection, the surgeon is cognizant of the possible existence of the non-recurrent, recurrent laryngeal nerve.

Throughout the thyroid surgery, and very often during this lateral dissection, many small blood vessels are encountered, which may be tied with suture ligature, cauterized with bipolar cautery, or cut with a harmonic scalpel.

The surgeon now directs his attention to the inferior pole. The surgeon isolates the inferior thyroid artery, but does not yet ligate it due to its close proximity to the recurrent laryngeal nerve. The recurrent laryngeal nerve supplies all of the intrinsic muscles of the larynx, except for the cricothyroid muscles, and is in contact with the posterior medial aspect of the thyroid gland, placing it at significant risk during thyroid surgery. Until the recurrent laryngeal nerve is located, blunt dissection only is used during inferior pole dissection. Most often, this nerve is located in a triangle between the trachea, the inferior pole of the thyroid, and the carotid artery. The surgeon performs blunt dissection with a Crile clamp and a Peanut Dissector. Locating the recurrent laryngeal nerve, which appears to be a white strand, he confirms the nerve's presence by touching it with an electrode which triggers a response in the nerve integrity monitor.

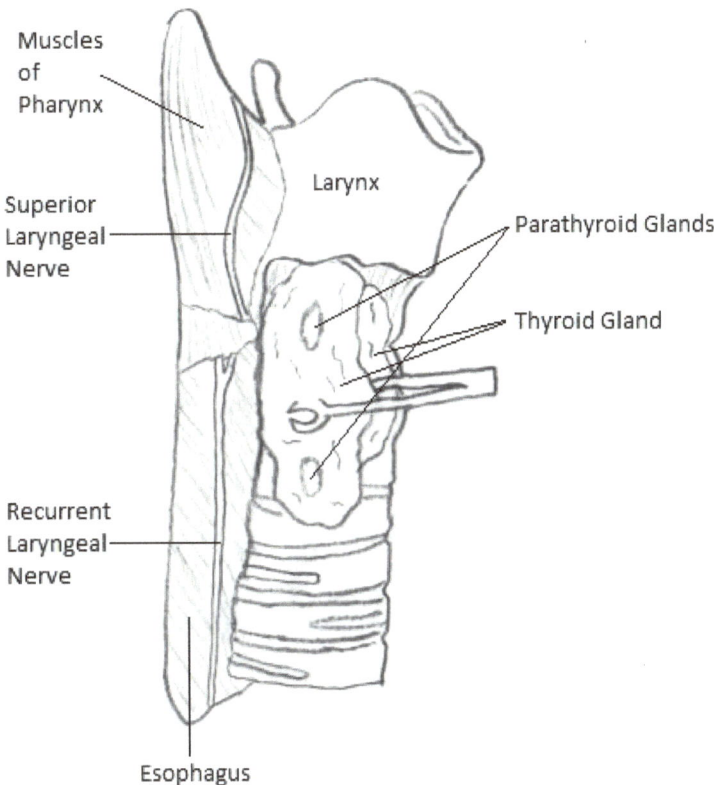

Fig.7.5. Anatomy of Neck Showing Recurrent Laryngeal Nerve.

7.7 THE OPERATION, PART 3: DISSECTING THE RECURRENT LARYNGEAL NERVE AND THYROID ISTHMUS. REMOVING THE RIGHT THYROID LOBE

With the nerve located, the surgeon directs his attention to the inferior thyroid artery and the nearby inferior parathyroid gland. The inferior thyroid artery is then double clamped along the inferior pole of the thyroid gland, incised, and ligated. The inferior parathyroid gland is then bluntly dissected away from the inferior pole, out of harm's way. Next, the thyroid isthmus is elevated off of the trachea with a Kelly clamp. The isthmus is then clamped in its entire length on both the right and left side with Kelly clamps and then incised and ligated.

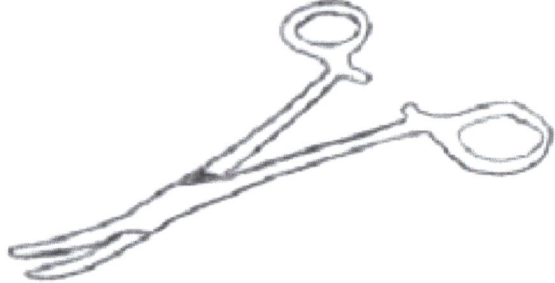

Fig.7.6. Kelly Clamp.

Attention is then redirected at the previously located recurrent laryngeal nerve inferiorly. Placing gentle inferior traction on the nerve using a moistened gauze pad, the surgeon dissects tissues off of the nerve using a Crile clamp in a superior direction. These tissues, including Berry's ligament, are then incised sharply, further exposing the nerve and releasing the thyroid lobe from its tracheal attachment. This process is continued until the nerve is seen to enter the larynx superiorly. Bleeders are often controlled during this step using a bipolar cautery.

The superior parathyroid gland is then found along the superior posterior surface of the thyroid. This gland, in addition to the remaining tissues binding the thyroid deeply, is sharply dissected and the right thyroid lobe is removed from the patient and sent to pathology.

7.8   THE OPERATION, PART 4: CONCLUSION

During the 15-20 minutes it takes for the pathologist to examine the nodule in question, the surgical bed is irrigated with sterile water and any bleeding vessels are localized and cauterized or tied off with sutures.

If pathology shows that the nodule is benign, which this chapter will assume it does, a drain is placed in the surgical bed, the wound is closed, and a dressing is applied. A drain is a tube used to prevent the accumulation of blood in the wound bed. The drain placed may be a closed system, which uses a vacuum bulb, or an open system, which acts as a wick and allows blood to seep into an overlying dressing.

If the pathology shows that the thyroid nodule is cancerous, the surgeon will often remove the remaining left thyroid lobe.

The wound is closed in layers. The platysma is re-approximated using absorbable sutures, followed by the subcutaneous tissues and then the skin. Most often, the skin is closed with a subcuticular non-absorbable stitch, which is removed 10 days post operatively. Certain glues have also been used for closure of the skin. A moderate pressure dressing is then applied with layers of thick gauze.

7.9   POST OPERATION

The patient is awakened and extubated after the operation and their vocal cords are examined. They are kept in the hospital overnight and so long as there has been only modest blood loss through the drain, the drain is then removed. The patient's ionized calcium level is checked to assure that there is acceptable parathyroid gland function. Thyroid hormone levels are checked in four weeks, as they take this long to show any significant change. If the thyroid function is low, thyroid hormone therapy is prescribed.

CHAPTER 8

PROCESS OF MEDICINE IN ARTHRITIS

Jason Guss

Rheumatologists are presented with a wide variety of patients complaining of pain, inflammation, and other widespread systemic effects. Arthritis is one of the primary diagnoses made by rheumatologists. There are several different types of arthritis, including osteoarthritis (mechanical), rheumatoid, psoriatic, and reactive. These different types of arthritis all have overlapping symptomology that can be misleading to the physician and can make correct diagnosis difficult. This chapter focuses on the process of medicine in arthritis and the correct diagnosis and treatment of mechanical and inflammatory arthritis types.

8.1 PATIENT HISTORY

The process of medicine begins with a detailed medical history of the patient. In musculoskeletal disorders, 80% of the diagnoses come from the patients' history [1]. The initial goal of the history and the physical exam is to identify if the arthritis is mechanical (osteoarthritis) or inflammatory. The history aims to evaluate several aspects of the medical problem. Initially, details of the chief complaint, such as location, duration, onset, pattern of joint involvement, and pain type, will be identified. Identification of joint involvement is important in diagnosis, as symmetry of location is indicative of rheumatoid arthritis (RA), whereas osteoarthritis typically begins on one side of the body. The onset and duration of the injury allows the physician to determine if the problem is a chronic issue or is the result of a single mechanical load. Osteoarthritis presents with more pain following activity and the primary complaint is typically pain. Inflammatory arthritis symptoms, on the other hand, frequently improve with physical activity and are commonly accompanied by morning stiffness and fatigue. The severity of the injury can be partially assessed by quantifying subsequent alterations in lifestyle. There are several health assessment questionnaires (HAQ) that are utilized to quantify the degree of one's symptoms and to measure the treatment outcome.

Next, one needs to learn of the patient's social, familial, and medical history. The social history may detail work and environmental factors that have influenced symptoms, as well as show how the patient's social interactions have been affected by the injury. The family history is another key component in the evaluation of arthritis, as it can show if there is a genetic predisposition to musculoskeletal system injury. Past medical history details previous medical treatment and medical ailments of the patient. It is important for the physician to examine the medical history in detail, as a patient may not disclose a past symptom due to disbelief that it is related to the current ailment.

The last primary component of the history is a review of all the major body systems (circulatory, respiratory, nervous, digestive, etc.). It is important to consider possible systemic disorders that could be related to the patient's complaints.

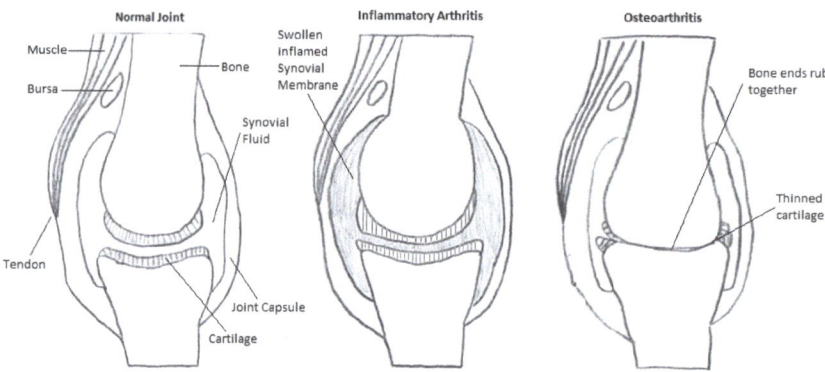

Fig.8.1. Normal Joint, Inflammatory Arthritis, Osteoarthritis

8.2   PHYSICAL EXAMINATION

The physical examination process helps the physician further evaluate the symptoms. If inflammatory arthritis is suspected based on the history, a more thorough examination of all joints should be conducted. However, if it appears that symptoms are acute and localized only to one primary location, a less comprehensive examination can be conducted, as mechanical arthritis is less systemic. During the physical exam, the physician will have the patient walk across the room so that a description of the gait can be recorded. Viewing the patient in a standing position allows the physician to identify possible abnormalities in the patient's posture, misalignment of the lower extremities, and disposition of the ankles or feet [1]. The physician examines the upper extremities to assess any abnormal contours, joint function, and identify other irregular findings. Joint function is determined by evaluating the range of limb motion, rotation of joints in all directions, and strength. Irregular findings are examined by inspection and palpation to identify any soft-tissue swelling, bursitis, nodules, or other disease manifestations [1].

Swelling can be assessed by holding one set of fingers stationary on a joint while simultaneously squeezing the joint with the other hand in order to detect potential fluid flow in an uncommon area. The lower extremities are assessed in a similar manner in order to evaluate for alignment issues, joint function, and other disease manifestations. During the physical examination, the physician typically assesses extra-articular features as well, as symptoms may present as rheumatoid nodules, nail changes, rashes, ulcers, and neurological abnormalities [1]. The patient's reflexes are also checked in order to assess any adverse neurological involvement related to the disease. Oftentimes, pain presenting in the lower extremities is the result of sciatica (pain related to the agitation of a sciatic nerve) and it is important to separate these symptoms from those caused by arthritis or other related injury. After taking a comprehensive history and physical examination, a physician should have a good indication of the cause of the patient's symptoms.

8.3   DIAGNOSTIC PROCEDURES

Following the history and medical exam, physicians have a variety of imaging tools and laboratory tests at their disposal to further evaluate the patient. X-ray imaging, which provides a clear picture of bone anatomy, calcification of soft tissues, and joint spacing, is typically the first imaging modality used [1]. Using X-ray imaging, a physician can easily identify a mechanical break in the bone, narrow joint spacing, and other mechanical related issues. Osteoporosis can also be identified with a radiograph based on the apparent density of the bone, but this is significantly more difficult. A limitation of X-ray imaging is that it does not effectively differentiate between the major types of soft tissue, such as muscle, ligaments, cartilage, and others. To identify abnormalities or problems with these tissues, a physician must use other imaging modalities. Magnetic Resonance Imaging (MRI) is a multi-planar imaging technique that is better suited to help identify problems with soft tissue. MRI is capable of identifying tears of muscle, tendons, and ligaments, as well as loss of cartilage and inflammation in the joint space [1]. MRI is often used to examine the patient if the patient's symptoms are suspected to relate to back and neck, as MRI can effectively visualize the nerves in this area. If these imaging modalities prove inconclusive, ultrasound may be used to further evaluate the issue. Because ultrasound reflects off bone, it is more useful for diagnosing soft tissue related problems, as opposed to skeletal. Ultrasound can effectively visualize tendons and check for damage, continuity, tears, and inflammation. Fluid appears black on ultrasound, which makes identifying extra fluid (inflammation) in a joint area somewhat easy for the physician. Ultrasound is also used for guidance of injections/aspirations because of its real time feedback and its ability to distinguish between soft tissues.

Various laboratory tests are also used by physicians to properly diagnose a patient. After taking the history and physical, the physician will decide which tests they deem important for confirming or ruling out certain pathologies. Due to the vast number of existing blood tests, only several important examples will be discussed here. A main goal of many laboratory tests is to determine if the symptoms are a result of inflammation. The erythrocyte sedimentation rate measure level of inflammation is one test to accomplish this. This test measures the rate of fall of red blood cells, which is useful because blood cells of those suffering from inflammation tend to form stacks and have a higher sedimentation rate [2]. Measuring the C-reactive protein (CRP) is another test to gauge the level of inflammation, as CRP levels rise during inflammatory processes [2]. These tests are non-specific to arthritis and other musculoskeletal problems, however, and positive tests do not confirm that the inflammation is related to a patient's arthritic disease. Autoantibodies are another category of markers that rheumatologists use in diagnosis. Rheumatoid factor is an immunoglobulin that is highly correlated with rheumatoid arthritis (present/elevated in 50-75% of cases), and therefore evaluation of rheumatoid factors can impact the diagnosis [1]. Anti-cyclic citrullinated peptide antibodies (anti-CCP) are also useful in diagnosing RA because these antibodies are found in the serum of patients with RA 40-70% of the time [1]. The measurement of anti-CCP can also serve as an important predictor of RA, as 93% of patients with undifferentiated arthritis who also have anti-CCP are found to later develop RA [1]. Antinuclear antibodies (ANA) are those that target proteins within the cell nucleus [2]. These antibodies are potential markers of autoimmune disease because they can label self-proteins as a target for the body to attack. Physicians also check for anemia because it is common for patients with inflammatory disease to have a low red blood cell count. Aspiration of a joint, in which the physician drains and examines joint fluid, is another diagnostic test at the physician's disposal. Joint aspiration is performed to check cell count, which is related to inflammation, and examine possible infection.

8.4   TREATMENT OPTIONS

Assuming a successful diagnosis is made, a physician must then focus on developing a treatment plan for the patient. The treatment plans for mechanical versus inflammatory arthritis can vary wildly. Oftentimes, if the OA is found early enough physical therapy is suggested, as therapy can strengthen nearby tendons, muscles, and ligaments to develop a support system for the weakened/damaged area. Weight loss may also be recommended if the patient is obese because the extra weight increases the load on the joints and can cause excess wear and tear. Similarly, lifestyle modifications may also be recommended if the patient is extremely active or participates in activities that put them at unnecessary risk. Another treatment option is the use of non-steroidal anti-inflammatory drugs (NSAIDs) that will provide pain relief, as well as mild anti-inflammatory effects [1]. Though NSAIDS reduce pain, they often do not improve the patient's outcome. Steroid injections are one of the last options for patients with bad OA and a considerable amount of inflammation before turning to surgical intervention. Cortisone is the steroid most commonly used and is a powerful anti-inflammatory that works to suppress the immune system in the injection area. This reduction of inflammation can also lead to temporary pain relief and improved joint function. If all of these options fail, surgical intervention is typically considered by the physician. With severe osteoarthritis, surgical intervention usually entails a joint replacement, as it is not possible to repair severe cartilage loss.

When upon diagnosis it is determined that the patient has inflammatory arthritis, other courses of treatment are pursued. A low-level anti-inflammatory, such as Advil, is usually tried first, as reduction of symptoms using Advil is preferable to the use of more serious drugs. If treatment with the low level anti-inflammatory is ineffective, Prednisone or another common corticosteroid is used, as these drugs suppress the immune system and can effectively treat autoimmune diseases. The next class of therapeutic drugs which is used if treatment is ineffective is disease modifying anti-rheumatic drugs (DMARD's). DMARD's are capable of reducing the progression of joint damage. Methotrexate is a preferred drug from this class, as it has shown to be effective for many years. Methotrexate alters T cell activation and expression, which limits the autoimmune response that the body mounts [3]. The new class of DMARD's that have emerged in recent years are called biologics. These are genetically engineered proteins that target specific components of the immune system to minimize its response [4]. Some examples of the major biologics prescribed are Adalimumab (Humira), Infliximab (Remicade), and Etanercept (Enbrel). Biologics have been proven very effective and in some patients can eliminate signs of the disease entirely. However, biologics should be avoided if the patient is immune compromised or currently has an infection, as the drugs target the TNF alpha pathway and reduce the immune system, leaving the patient more susceptible to these risks [4].

CHAPTER 9

PHARMACEUTICALS IN MEDICINE

Andrew Luzzi and Martin Prince MD

Use of chemicals, aka "pharmaceuticals" or "drugs" or "agents" to treat disease is a major backbone of the practice of medicine. For many diseases, options for treatment are commonly categorized into surgical options or medical options where "medical treatment" is generally referring to the clever choice of the right pharmaceutical agents to make the disease go away. However, even for surgical options, treatment of the diseases always needs to be supports of pharmaceuticals. Huge texts compile the vast array of drugs which are FDA approved for use in treating diseases and even more agents can be found "off-the-shelf" at pharmacies or health food stores. One popular book, known as Physicians' Desk Reference is provided free to all doctors and clinics. This ubiquitous text has one index based on the generic names, a second index based on trade names, a third index based upon the drug categories (more on this below) and a fourth index showing the shape and color of each pill so that patients can tell you what they are taking even if they do not speak English or know the name of the drug.

It is beyond the scope of an introduction to pharmaceuticals to begin delving into specific pharmaceuticals. However, it is useful to understand the categories of pharmaceutical agents which are available and to know the process of how specific agents are chosen as well as how the dose and duration of treatment are titrated to match the needs of individual patients.

9.1   ANTIBIOTICS

These are miracle drugs that can restore a person on their deathbed to normal health in short order. Hundreds of choices reflect the many different organisms which can cause infection and destruction of human tissues. Antibiotics are drugs which are used for bacterial infection. A rigorous approach for reasonably healthy patients with mild infection, not yet life threatening, is the "No bug, No drug" rule. In this approach, the infected area is swabbed or aspirated so that the bacteria can be cultured, e.g. grown on petri dishes with agar. Once the bacteria grow, small discs of various antibiotics are placed on the infested agar to determine which antibiotic is the most effective at treating that patient's infection. This antibiotic is then prescribed for the patient. Oral pills are the most tolerated but intravenous and intramuscular injection are more effective. Surface infection on the skin may be treated with an antibiotic cream.

Unfortunately, many patients/physicians are in a hurry and do not want to wait for the culture/drug sensitivity analysis to be completed. In this case, the antibiotic is chosen empirically based upon knowing the bacteria which most commonly cause that particular infection. With the empiric approach, a broad spectrum antibiotic is used, which kills a broad spectrum of bacteria in case the guess about the type of infecting one is not perfect. However, this has the disadvantage of also killing more of the patients' normal flora. Normal flora are bacteria and other microorganisms that are on the patient and in the intestines which help protect against nastier microbes as well as help with digestion and other processes.

9.2   ANTI-INFLAMMATORY

Anti-inflammatory drugs, as one would expect, reduce inflammatory processes in the body. Inflammation is a natural bodily response to trauma and other stimuli. Inflammation can be beneficial, as it promotes the flow of blood and immune cells to areas where they are needed for healing or immune defense, such as areas where the body has experienced injury and disruption that allows pathogens to invade into the body. However, inflammation typically also causes pain and too much inflammation may negatively affect disease/injury treatment and healing. When there has been only minor injury with no breach of the protective skin, an anti-inflammatory drug can help prevent the body from over-reacting.

Various kinds of anti-inflammatory drugs reduce the redness, swelling, and pain associated with inflammation. Corticosteroids are produced naturally by humans in the adrenal cortex and, among many other effects, regulate inflammation. Synthetic corticosteroids are used to treat inflammatory processes that are more systemic in nature, such as arthritis, allergies, and inflammatory bowel disease. Non-steroidal anti-inflammatory drugs (NSAIDs), are another main category of anti-inflammatory medication. Over the counter (OTC) NSAIDs, such as aspirin and ibuprofen (Advil, Motrin), are used to treat a wide range of inflammatory processes ranging from arthritis to sore muscles to inflammation resulting from injury.

9.3   PAINKILLERS (ANALGESICS)

While anti-inflammatory drugs reduce pain by reducing inflammatory processes, other drugs, commonly referred to as pain killers, reduce pain by directly affecting the central nervous system. The most powerful prescription painkillers are called opioids, which are opium-like compounds that affect the opioid receptors in our brains and, in so doing, decrease a patient's perception of pain and increase tolerance to pain.

Opioids can be injected into patients intravenously or taken by patients orally. The method of administration of the drug, as well as the dose and specific type of drug, depends on what is causing the patient pain. Opioids may be administered intravenously to patients with severe acute pain, such as pain arising from a sickle cell crisis or abdominal pain stemming from a ruptured appendix or myocardial infarction. Patients are often prescribed opioids to be taken orally in order to manage chronic pain, which can stem from a variety of causes, and post-operative pain.

However, opioid use can have adverse effects. Patients using opioids often experience nausea, drowsiness, and constipation. Additionally, opioids are physically addicting. Therefore, healthcare providers must be careful both to administer safe doses of drugs and also recognize and discourage drug seeking behavior.

There are many different pain medicines, and each one has advantages and risks. OTC pain relievers are good for many types of pain. There are two main types of OTC pain medicines: acetaminophen (Tylenol) and nonsteroidal anti-inflammatory drugs (NSAIDs). Aspirin, naproxen (Aleve), and ibuprofen (Advil, Motrin) are examples of OTC NSAIDs.

9.4   LOCAL ANESTHETICS

Local anesthetics are drugs that induce temporary lack of sensation in one part of the body. Various techniques and drugs exist to induce local anesthesia, and the specific method of induction is determined by the desired outcome of the medication.

Topical anesthetics, which are one category of local anesthetics, are applied to a body surface and, by increasing the excitability threshold of the nerves in that area, numb local tissue. Topical anesthetics exist in many forms and have a wide range of applications. Cream can be applied to an arm to numb the skin before the administration of an IV, spray can be used to numb the throat before the insertion of a scope, liquid can be applied via cotton swab to the mouth before the administration of an injectable anesthetic prior to dental work, and other forms of topical anesthetic and methods of administration exist and are used for a wide range of purposes.

Nerve blocks are another broad category of local anesthetic use. Unlike topical anesthetics, which are generally applied to and affect superficial tissue, nerve blocks involve the direct injection of an anesthetic, among several other drugs, onto a nerve. In so doing, entire parts of the body, such as limbs and joints, can be relieved of sensation, resulting in less pain during certain procedures and surgeries.

A third category of local anesthetic use is epidural anesthesia. With epidural anesthesia, an anesthetic is injected into the epidural space around the spinal cord in order to numb different parts of the body. Epidural anesthesia is commonly used to provide pain relief during labor and delivery and is also commonly used to provide pain relief during operations on the lower part of the body.

9.5   GENERAL ANESTHETICS

While local anesthetics are used to numb different parts of the body, general anesthetics are drugs that induce unconsciousness in patients. They are commonly used during more intensive and/or uncomfortable operations so that the patient does not feel any pain during the procedure or have any memory of the procedure after its completion. Under general anesthesia, patients also experience skeletal muscle relaxation which can make surgery easier.

General anesthetics are just one part of general anesthesia. Anesthesia refers to the coma-like state into which patients are induced for various reasons. The induction and maintenance of patients into a state of anesthesia is a complicated process that involves the simultaneous administration of several drugs, including sedatives, paralytics, pain killers, general anesthetics, and often others. General anesthetics can be administered through an IV or as vapors using a mask.

Various measures must be taken to ensure the safety of the patient while under general anesthesia. A physician or registered nurse monitors the administration of drugs throughout the procedure, in addition to monitoring the vital signs (heart rate, respiratory rate, temperature and blood pressure) of the patient. Also, because of the depressing effects of the anesthesia medication, patients are unable to breathe for themselves. Various methods of mechanical ventilation exist to assist the breathing of the patient while under general anesthesia.

9.6   MUSCLE RELAXANTS

Muscle relaxants are drugs that act to decrease muscle contraction and relax muscles. Most muscle relaxants are referred to as "centrally acting". This means that they reduce muscular contraction by increasing the inhibitory signals sent to motor neurons by the central nervous system. These drugs are used to treat various conditions, many having to do with muscle spasms and muscle pain. Muscle relaxants are typically taken orally.

Because of their depressive effects on the central nervous system, muscle relaxants often induce fatigue and lethargy in patients. Nausea, vomiting, and other more rare side effects can also result from the use of muscle relaxants. Additionally, muscle relaxants have the potential to be abused for recreational purposes and patients occasionally become addicted. Both physicians and patients must be aware of this possibility and take measures to prevent dependence.

9.7   ANTI-ANXIETY (ANXIOLYTIC)

Benzodiazepines are a class of drugs categorized by a similar fundamental structure that have general anti-anxiety, sleep-inducing, muscle relaxing, and calming effects. The drugs work by enhancing the function of a neurotransmitter in the brain in order to decrease the excitability of neurons. In doing so, benzodiazepines are used to treat panic disorders, anxiety disorders, and some cases of insomnia.

Like muscle relaxants, anxiolytic benzodiazepines also pose significant risk for abuse. Patients using anxiolytic benzodiazepines naturally develop a tolerance, and some patients will increase their drug use in order to receive the same effects from the drugs. It is possible to become dependent on anxiolytic benzodiazepines and go through withdrawal when usage stops.

9.8   CHEMOTHERAPY

Chemotherapy treatments use cytotoxic drugs – or drugs that are toxic to living cells – to help cancer patients fight their disease. The cytotoxic drugs in chemotherapy are optimized to destroy rapidly multiplying cells occurring in cancer. Chemotherapy is administered in a variety of ways, including orally, topically, with the use of an injection, through an IV, and more. This method can successfully kill cancer cells, which are rapidly multiplying, and subsequently slow or stop cancer growth and alleviate cancer symptoms. However, the drugs also have a cytotoxic effect on healthy cells, which results in a wide range of adverse effects for the patient. Because of this, chemotherapy treatment is often given in cycles, allowing rest time so that the patient's body can recuperate and rebuild healthy cells that were killed during treatment.

Even with incorporated rest time during chemotherapy treatment, patients who are undergoing treatment experience a spectrum of side effects. As stated, chemotherapy drugs target rapidly dividing cells. Hair follicle cells, bone marrow cells, and cells in the digestive tract are all non-cancerous rapidly dividing cells that are typically affected by chemotherapy treatment. As such, patients undergoing chemotherapy typically experience hair loss, a decrease in blood cell production, and inflammation of the mucosal lining. Chemotherapy also typically induces nausea, vomiting, and fatigue in cancer patients, along with a variety of other adverse effects.

9.9   CARDIAC DRUGS

Normal functioning of the cardiovascular system is critical to human life to ensure oxygen delivery to the brain and other organs. When a patient is critically ill and the cardiovascular system is no longer functioning properly, there are a host of pharmaceuticals (referred to as cardiac drugs) that can influence different components of this system to keep the patient alive long enough for recovery. There is a delicate balance between the pumping of the heart and the resistance in the arterioles throughout the body. During sepsis, arterioles relax, decreasing peripheral vascular resistance, causing the blood pressure to drop. To compensate, the heart needs to pump faster and more vigorously. But in many patients, the heart is already maxed out and cannot pump any harder. Epinephrine (also known as adrenaline), can stimulate the heart rate, the heart pumping power, known as inotropy, and can cause peripheral vascular arteriolar constriction to increase peripheral vascular resistance. This has the effect of increasing blood pressure. Epinephrine can also dilate bronchioles which is useful to treat allergic reactions causing bronchoconstriction.

Elements of the cardiovascular system may be controlled by alpha receptors or beta receptors. Alpha receptors mediate vasoconstriction, so drugs stimulating the alpha receptors cause vasoconstriction and raise the blood pressure. Beta receptors cause vasorelaxation and bronchodilation, so compounds that activate beta receptors cause vasodilation and lower blood pressure. Beta blockers will slow the heart rate and decrease the cardiac workload, giving the heart a rest. Beta blockers also prevent dramatic increases in heart rate due to stress, so some people use these prior to important lectures or phobic experiences. Beta 1 receptors also mediate increased cardiac output by increasing heart rate and inotropy. Beta 2 receptors mediate bronchodilation and thus beta 2 agonists are better for treating asthma and allergic reactions.

There are many pharmaceuticals which are very selective, primarily affecting only 1 element of the cardiovascular system. Hydralazine, for example, primarily causes decreased peripheral vascular resistance and can be useful for rapidly treating malignant hypertension.

9.10   HORMONE REPLACEMENT THERAPY

When an organ fails or needs to be removed, the functioning of that organ may be replaced by taking the compounds produced by that organ in the form of a pill. For example, if the thyroid gland has a suspicious nodule and is surgically removed, the patient will then have low thyroid hormone levels. This can be corrected by taking thyroxine once a day. After many bouts of pancreatitis, the destroyed pancreas will no longer produce digestive enzymes. These can then be taken orally with each meal. The islet cells in the pancreas, which produce insulin, may be destroyed, requiring the patient to take regular doses of insulin. Without insulin, fat, muscle and other cells will not transport sugar in the blood into the cell. The cells are starving and the patient is hyperglycemic. High viscosity, hyperglycemic blood gradually destroys the blood vessels, creating havoc throughout the entire patient. Older women produce less estrogen, especially after menopause. Estrogen replacement therapy preserves bone density, stabilizes menopause symptoms, e.g. hot flashes, and restores a premenopausal status to female reproductive tissues. But a side effect of estrogen replacement therapy is increased breast cancer and endometrial cancer risk, so it must be used cautiously. Other examples of hormone replacements include pituitary, adrenal, and androgens. Patients undergoing gender conversions may use hormones to alter their physical appearance, and athletes may use androgens to boost their athletic performance.

www.ingramcontent.com/pod-product-compliance
Lightning Source LLC
Chambersburg PA
CBHW050723180526
45159CB00003B/1115